PAIN: A FOUR-LETTER WORD YOU CAN LIVE WITH

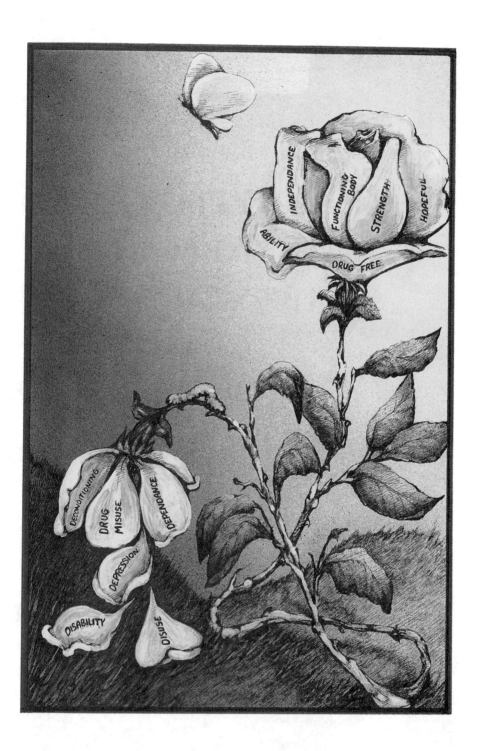

PAIN: A FOUR-LETTER WORD YOU CAN LIVE WITH

Sridhar V. Vasudevan, M.D.

Pain: A Four-Letter Word You Can Live With
Sridhar V. Vasudevan, M.D.

ISBN 0-929867-05-7

Set in Goudy and Stone Sans by Montgomery Media, Inc.
Cover design by Montgomery Media, Inc.
Printed and bound by BookCrafters
Illustrations by Mary Crockett

Printed in the United States of America

*This book is not intended as a substitute for the medical advice of
physicians. Before attempting any of the exercises described herein,
please speak with your doctor. The reader should regularly consult a
physician in matters relating to his or her health but particularly with
respect to any symptoms that may require specific medical attention or
medication. The names of patients used in this book have been changed
to protect their identity.*

This book is dedicated to my parents

Mr. S. Vasudevan
and
Mrs. Rukimini Vasudevan

who instilled in me my basic value system
and provided me with unconditional love.

CONTENTS

FOREWORD

C hronic pain has achieved epidemic proportions in the industrialized nations. Disability due to chronic pain is one of the major health care and compensation costs in the United States. Low back pain alone has been estimated to cost the country over $50 billion every year. Although many consider this to be a medical problem, it is quite obvious that chronic pain extends beyond the medical realm into the political, social, and economic lives of our citizens. Traditional health care, based on a biomedical model, is often one of the causes rather than remedies for chronic pain. Fortunately, there is a small number of physicians and health care organizations that recognize the unique characteristics of chronic pain patients. They utilize a bio-psycho-social concept of illness that is far more effective in restoring patients to wellness.

One of the leaders in the movement has been Dr. Sridhar Vasudevan. In this book he describes the problems that plague patients with chronic pain. The book is based upon his observations and experiences and is aimed at the chronic pain patient. Reading and learning the concepts espoused by Dr. Vasudevan will start a chronic pain patient on the road to recovery. Self-help alone rarely solves the problem, but an informed consumer who understands the issues addressed in the management of chronic pain is more likely to profit from a pain treatment program. I recommend this book to the chronic pain sufferer who wishes to embark upon the journey to the road of better functioning and less pain.

In addition to explaining how the body works, Dr. Vasudevan has identified the important features of pain treatment programs. The book offers a balanced perspective that does not make inappropriate claims for miraculous cures that are so common in self-help and medical information books. This book is written by an insider who clearly knows the problems that chronic pain sufferers endure. He also knows the ingredients of a successful pain management program. This is an excellent resource and should be available in public libraries, as well as primary care practitioners' offices.

John D. Loeser, M.D.
Professor, Neurological Surgery & Anesthesiology
Director, Multidisciplinary Pain Center
University of Washington, Seattle, WA

---

*T*he usual doctor treats disease, the good doctor treats ailments, the rare doctor treats the person. Dr. Vasudevan is such a rare doctor. His book embodies his commitment to treating the person, which is essential to the successful rehabilitation of chronic pain disability. In plain language, he methodically leads the reader to recognize the nature of chronic pain disability and then instructs and illustrates how one participates in lessening the disability.

For understanding the experience of chronic pain and its treatment, this book is an excellent primer for patients, their families, third-party insurance carriers, and government regulators. Public libraries would profit their members by stocking the book, while professionals would benefit their patients by having them read it.

Peter J. Vicente, Ph.D.
President-Elect
American Pain Society

S ridhar Vasudevan, M.D., a leader in the field of chronic pain management, has provided you with a book to motivate you to receive appropriate help. This book can also be used by individuals who are enrolled in a chronic pain treatment program to reinforce the concepts of the program. Family members and friends can use this book to understand the concept of chronic pain and the difficulties an individual with chronic pain has to endure, and as a guide to support and help individuals through a pain program. Lastly, this book can also be used by health care professionals as a handout or suggested reading for people entering, participating in, and completing a pain treatment program.

I found this book well-written, easy to read, and understandable for the average person with chronic pain. The case scenarios before and the summaries at the end of each chapter puts each concept into perspective.

As Dr. Vasudevan says, "an appropriate pain treatment program can give you control over your pain rather than letting pain control you." This book helps you with that concept and will give insight and support to accomplish that goal.

Good luck and good reading.

Martin Grabois, M.D.
Professor and Chairman
Department of Physical Medicine and Rehabilitation
Baylor College of Medicine
Director, The Methodist Hospital Pain Management
Program
Houston, TX

C hronic illness can be a devastating situation for the person so affected. Unlike a broken bone, which mends in a matter of weeks or even heart disease, which can be effectively treated and recover with time, there is no definable "endpoint" for chronic illness. This is even more of a problem if chronic pain is the issue. With this condition, the patient and physician usually are dealing with symptoms not accompanied by any objective measurable physical findings that correlate to the pain.

Pain is an essential sensation, and while never pleasant, usually acts as a warning that there is actual or possible damage to tissue. The absence of pain can lead to serious bodily harm. On the other hand, pain without cause can lead to terrible suffering and neglect of personal and family responsibilities. Enormous psychological, vocational, and social issues arise in individuals experiencing long-standing chronic pain. This book addresses those factors and their impact on an individual's functional ability.

Dr. Vasudevan not only has been a leader in the professional chronic pain movement, but also has been actively involved in the treatment and management of patients afflicted by this disorder. While an active advocate for his patients, he has attempted to educate them in the biopsychosocial phenomena which constitute the chronic pain syndrome.

This book is a distillation of the psychological techniques and physical therapies Dr. Vasudevan and his team apply to their patients. It offers an explanation to patients and family, referring physicians as well as insurance representatives, as to the nature of the process required in treating chronic pain patients. The advice given here will enable a patient to begin to understand the necessity of his or her involvement in the rehabilitation process. It also enables the insurer to understand the complex psychological issues implicit in the chronic pain syndrome and the intensity and diversity of therapies required to treat it.

This self-help book can be invaluable to the chronic pain patient and his or her family or support source. Especially with professional guidance, he or she can easily begin the behavioral, cognitive, and physical modifications essential to restructuring of a pain-centered, nonproductive life. Even independently, the pain patient will see the wisdom of relinquishing an unfulfilling lifestyle in order to resume a more gratifying life. I am sure that the patient, family, and pain professional alike will find this to be an invaluable aid in dealing with chronic pain, and I plan to make it required reading for my patients.

E. Richard Blonsky, M.D.
Director, Center for Pain Studies
Rehabilitation Institute of Chicago
Past President, American Academy
of Pain Medicine

D r. Sridhar Vasudevan has approached the difficult and complex problem of chronic pain with a straightforward and practical program. His book, *Pain: a Four-Letter Word You Can Live With*, is based on his wide experience as a specialist in pain medicine and rehabilitation. It contains information and insights that will be invaluable to those patients suffering with chronic pain. The techniques he describes will be of great benefit to such individuals, and should help them maximize their function and enjoyment. The same issues are also of great importance to the friends and relatives of patients in pain in dealing with the inevitable personal, social, and vocational disruptions. The book will also be of great interest and assistance to physicians and other health care professionals, who tend to deal with the technology and bureaucracy of pain management instead of the personal aspects. The concepts contained in the book will improve relationships between the patient and the helpers. In short, Dr. Vasudevan has successfully addressed important issues for pain patients, their families, and their health professionals in a book that will be invaluable for all of them.

Peter R. Wilson, M.B.B.S., Ph.D.
Consultant in Pain Medicine, Mayo Clinic
President, American Academy of Pain Medicine

Chronic pain disrupts the lives of more than 50 million Americans every year. Aside from the personal suffering of the patients with chronic pain, the cost to the American economy is staggering, amounting to more than $80 billion each year. These alarming statistics are made worse by the fact that proper treatment techniques for patients with chronic pain exist but are not frequently used.

Dr. Vasudevan, in his easily-readable and comprehensive book, addresses everything that the chronic pain sufferer needs to know to find the appropriate treatment for his/her suffering. This book should inspire hope and optimism that in spite of chronic pain, a productive, satisfying life can still be achieved with the appropriate help.

Norman Marcus, M.D.
Director, New York Pain Treatment Program
Lenox Hill Hospital, New York

PREFACE

A book about having dreams . . . and making them come true

In many ways, this book is about dreams—dreams of being whole again, dreams of living life to the fullest, dreams of being the best you can be. I know about dreams because this book is the realization of a longtime dream of mine—to write a book about managing chronic pain, a book based on my experience with patients with pain. I have seen such miraculous results with my patients that I want to share their experiences and approaches with others suffering this seemingly endless, purposeless pain that can destroy people's lives—the kind of pain that is called *chronic pain*.

Almost all of my patients have said to me something like, "Dr. V., what this program did was give me control over my pain rather than letting the pain control me." It is my great hope that with this book I can help readers gain this kind of control over their pain and their lives.

Throughout the book, I have incorporated the personal accounts and experiences of my patients. Though statistics recounted in the book reflect the magnitude of the problem of chronic pain, we must remember that these hard numbers represent real people who could be your relatives, your neighbors or yourself.

Purpose of this book

I have written this book for individuals who, like my patients, have had pain for many months or even years, and who have sought many kinds of treatment, including narcotic medications, physical therapy, surgery, or other treatments which have essentially failed. Many times, these people have gone from doctor to doctor searching with no success for a diagnosis and a cure. The point at which these people come to me (or the point at which you may have started to read this book) is when there seems to be no hope—perhaps when a doctor has thrown up his hands and said that there is nothing more that can be done about this pain.

The book is also written for the families of these people—family members who are at a loss about how to deal with someone who seems to have given up on life because of pain that is difficult for anyone else to understand. Family members can play an extremely important role in helping the person manage pain, and that role may be just the opposite of what the family member feels is his or her responsibility. It may mean not doing everything for the person in pain. It may mean directing attention away from that person. It may mean enabling a person to manage his or her own life instead of being dependent on a caregiver. These can be very difficult steps for a family member to take. This book offers information and advice to help in determining if these steps are necessary and then taking them.

Just as I do not have exact answers or guarantees of permanent pain relief for my patients, I do not have them for readers of this book. But I do promise to help guide you in learning to understand chronic pain and function with more control despite it.

Chronic pain—a complex devastating process

Over the last fifteen years I've had the opportunity to see and participate in the rehabilitation of more than 5,000 individuals with pain. Most of these people have had chronic and persistent pain which had not responded to previous approaches to treatment. These have included a variety of approaches including medications, surgical interventions, chiropractic care, physical therapy, and other treatments—none of which helped these individuals gain control over their pain. Constant pain had become the compelling force in their lives, incapacitating them from carrying on their usual daily roles as workers, parents, spouses or homemakers.

These individuals had become dependent on medications, despite the fact that they frequently spoke of medications not being helpful. They continued to seek further evaluations and treatments which only led to further despondency and failure. Many of these individuals were eventually helped through the approaches discussed in this book.

I too, at a very personal level, have experienced the disabling results of chronic pain. Since my early teenage years, I've had headaches. These would occur initially only occasionally but soon became a daily problem. Evaluations revealed that I required glasses and corrective lenses were prescribed. Although this did help some aspects of the headaches, the severe throbbing continued over the next several years. After seeing many physicians, I was diagnosed as having migraine headaches. I tried most of the usual medications, but relief was only temporary.

As I pursued my medical school and residency training, these headaches continued, varying in intensity. Relatives, friends and medical colleagues suggested different treatments and soon I found myself using a variety of medications. Finally, after a brain scan and other attempts at diagnosis revealed no significant medical problem, a friendly physician advised that I try approaches other than drugs. So, I started stretching exercises and attempted to control as much of the stress in my life as possible. Now, when the headaches do occur, I don't search for complete relief or a "cure," but instead try various diverting, stress-relieving techniques which move my focus away from the headaches.

With the advances made by research into headaches, it is clear that there are hundreds of reasons for them. Recognizing the stresses that provoke the headaches and trying to avoid them, using non-addictive medications for severe headaches, and applying the psychological principles discussed in this book, I've been able to continue my career in rehabilitation medicine. I am now able to fulfill my role as a physician and my dreams of having a family, caring for my patients, and teaching the concepts I've learned about pain management.

Pain—a personal experience

Pain is an intensely personal experience. No one can understand it completely but the person who has it. No one can determine its intensity but that person. And no one can learn how to manage it but the person who experiences it. The attitude with which you approach pain is yours. You can decide to give up or you can decide to move forward. You can decide to dwell on your pain today with no hope for the future—or you can decide that you do not want to be in the same condition tomorrow and do something about it. The decision is yours. *You do have a choice*. This book is designed to give you the *information, resources and confidence* to make the necessary changes that will allow you to live a productive, happy life. The major point I make to my patients and want to make to you, the readers of this book, is that you can control pain. When you realize this, you have taken the essential first step toward managing your pain.

In the last thirty years, significant advances have been made in the understanding and treatment of chronic pain. The next several decades, in my opinion, will produce an even better understanding of the neurochemical basis of pain. Advances in better diagnosis, as well as better medications should become available. However, pain has been in existence since prehistoric times and will probably continue to exist in the future. This is because pain is more than a purely physical phenomenon. You will learn that the experience of pain not only involves biological processes in our bodies but includes psychological, social and environmental factors. Some of these are beyond your control. However, you can control your response to these events with proper training and knowledge.

Chronic pain is a crisis in a person's life. However, *as is the case with other crises, out of pain may come opportunity*—opportunity for reevaluation, for refocusing, for generating new energy and new commitment. I have seen patients come into my office almost completely disabled, perhaps in wheelchairs or grimacing with every movement. Several weeks later, after applying the principles they have learned in a pain rehabilitation program, they are moving with ease. More importantly, they may have made choices in their lives that they never would have considered before.

One patient decides to go back to college. Another makes a firm commitment to a marriage that had at one point seemed beyond repair. Another develops a new dedication and excitement about his career. I often wonder if these positive steps would have been taken if these people had not faced the crisis of their pain and been forced to reevaluate almost every aspect of their lives.

A problem-solving attitude is very important in chronic pain management. Those who have solved problems are those who have persevered. As with most challenges in life, *quick fixes don't work.* When patients come to me expecting immediate cures, I know they will be disappointed. Impatience most often leads to failure.

To these patients, I cite examples of famous people throughout history who only found success through perseverance and patience. Darwin took a whole lifetime to develop his theory of evolution. Webster's dictionary took twenty-four years to create. Randolph Hearst writes of having thirty-six rejections of the first article he submitted for publication and yet he became a communications giant. Beethoven wrote his first major piece twenty times before he was satisfied, and Edison tried his light bulb ten thousand times before it worked. If these people had given up on their dreams, they never would have accomplished their goals.

The first step for you is to have a dream. Have a dream of controlling your pain and going on with your life, and then don't give up. Keep in mind that your ability to dream and hope for the future is affected by your own limitations. These limitations may have been learned through life experiences or forced on you by well-meaning family members or healthcare professionals. What may have seemed impossible for a long time may become possible if you make a commitment and start to believe you can accomplish your dream.

I remember well an elderly woman who was one of my patients. Crippled by arthritis, she was wheeled into my office in a wheelchair. She only hoped to relieve her pain and never even considered that she might walk again. By the end of three weeks in our pain rehabilitation program, she was literally bouncing up and down the halls in tennis shoes and a sweatsuit—all because she was inspired to dream again and to believe in herself. Such seeming miracles are not always possible; however, the possibility that they can happen should be an inspiration to anyone experiencing chronic pain.

Sometimes learning to dream again may mean breaking down some preconceived barriers. The four-minute mile is a good example of one such barrier. For years, four minutes was assumed to be the top speed in which a human being could run a mile. No one challenged this assumption until 1954. A young Englishman, Dr. Roger Gilbert Bannister, made up his mind that he could break this record and did it. He ran the mile on a track in Oxford in 3 minutes and 59.4 seconds. Now this barrier is broken consistently.

Though you may not come close to the four-minute mile, you may discover unbelievable possibilities within yourself by applying some of the principles outlined in this book. Some of you may be able to achieve your goals on your own and others may need the support of a "coach," who works closely with you and understands your potential and your limitations. This coach may be an understanding physician or the entire staff involved in a pain rehabilitation program. Later chapters offer guidance on choosing these coaches.

This book will emphasize some new concepts. Most of us are trained and conditioned by society to believe the following four common assumptions:

1. *Pain indicates that something is wrong.*

2. *Pain always has a cause which you can discover.*

3. *Pain means that there is a condition which can be cured.*

4. *After pain is resolved, you should be able to return to your normal functioning.*

These assumptions are true for most patients experiencing acute pain (for instance, after surgery or injury). In such situations, physicians and other healthcare providers usually do a marvelous job of diagnosing and treating pain, but they are not true for most chronic pain patients. These patients need to learn the following four new rules:

1. *Pain does not always indicate an underlying problem that needs to be diagnosed and treated.*

2. *Even when we know the cause of pain, there may be no proof by x-rays, blood tests, or other medical tests.*

3. *Even when an exact cause of pain can be proven, there is no permanent "cure" for the condition producing pain.*

4. *However, pain does not have to control your life just because it cannot be completely cured. With sufficient information and skills that can be learned, YOU CAN GAIN CONTROL OVER YOUR LIFE and return to being productive.*

Throughout this book, you will learn the how, why, what and when as they relate to pain. *Pain* as many of you may realize is a FOUR-letter word. Just like other four-letter words that convey an unpleasant and distasteful feeling, pain can be a significant negative four-letter word. However, through this book you learn that pain can be a useful symptom of an underlying disorder.

You'll also be exposed to other four-letter words that are positive, such as LOVE, WORK, and HOPE. Using the same theme, I have attempted to discuss many of the concepts with four-letter word titles. Thus, you'll be informed about the BELL and GATE theories of pain. You will learn the appropriate use of DRUG, implications of pain on WORK, and how to LIVE your life with optimal functioning without the use of medications. A TEAM approach is needed to accomplish the control over pain and the composition and the roles of such a team will be described.

I've always felt that knowledge is the best weapon and ignorance is not bliss. Therefore, this book emphasizes my philosophy of pain management which provides appropriate information and skills to those of you affected by pain so you can deal with its consequences. Then, using your own inner resources, you can effectively apply this information to your individual situations.

About this book

This book provides you with information that is both valuable and useful. Each of these chapters can stand by itself; however, if you are facing a disabling chronic pain problem you will probably eventually want to read the entire book because you will be dealing with almost every issue raised. I have tried to organize the material in a logical sequence. In the first chapter, the magnitude of the problem is presented along with the idea that pain impacts on every aspect of a person's life and family. In the second chapter, pain is defined with an emphasis on its complexities and the differences between chronic and acute pain. The third chapter is probably the most technical because it explains the various theories of pain with the goal of helping you understand how and why pain works in such seemingly mysterious ways. In the fourth chapter, we look at Chronic Benign Pain Syndrome, the combination of symptoms and characteristics which are so common in the person experiencing chronic pain.

The fifth chapter details the many different effective approaches for managing and living with chronic pain. In the sixth chapter we look at the team of professionals who frequently play an important role in pain management. In the seventh chapter we discuss the essential process of integrating pain management into your life. The eighth chapter presents discussions of how to evaluate success from pain programs. The final chapter emphasizes living with hope and optimism and setting lifetime goals. The appendix offers many useful resources which supplement this book by providing further information and insights.

Each chapter begins with a description of a patient seen commonly in a pain rehabilitation center. The names are not real, but these examples reflect a composite of individuals (like you) who I have seen and cared for in my practice. Many of these patients eventually participated in the pain rehabilitation center and regained control over their pain and their lives.

This book is full of dreams and hopes—my dreams and those of my patients. If you or a loved one is experiencing pain, you may recognize your dreams here too. If you are helped, then my dream is fulfilled. Hippocrates said, "Physicians cure a few, help many, but comfort all." You may be comforted by the fact that you are not alone. You will also learn that others, in similar situations, have been able to have an open mind and understand the major concepts of chronic pain management which are explained in this book.

What works for one person may not work for another. In this book, we will discuss many effective techniques for dealing with pain. Each individual needs to find the approach or combination of techniques which works best for him/her. Some people find biofeedback effective while others realize that a daily walk produces the same good results. Some people find encouragement in group support sessions while others would rather work one-on-one with a psychologist. Some people do both. Some do neither and are still successful. An inpatient pain program may be the answer for you while another person may be able to apply effective pain management principles on an outpatient basis. The path to your dream of leading a full life and handling your pain may be different, but the point is—have a dream, learn about possible paths to take, and then apply the principles outlined in this book!

In summary, my wish for you is that this book will help you understand and control your pain and your life. It may help if you keep in mind what Confucius said centuries ago:

I hear and I forget.
I see and I remember.
I do and I understand.

Wishing you success and the best of health,
Sridhar V. Vasudevan, M.D.
Milwaukee, Wisconsin

ACKNOWLEDGMENTS

I wish to acknowledge the following individuals, without whose support my dream of this book would not have become reality.

Doreen, my wife, for her constant friendship and encouragement of my activities.

John and *Michael*, my sons, who provide meaning to my life.

Raj, my brother, who has always shown confidence in me and has provided constant encouragement and support.

Tim Lynch, Ph.D., a supportive friend and colleague, for his encouragement and contributions to the book regarding stress management.

Mrs. Joan Zizzo, my secretary, and *Mrs. Mary Reich*, nurse clinician, for their loyal and dedicated support of my practice.

Susan Montgomery, who assisted in turning my ideas and concepts into a readable book; also the staff associated with Montgomery Media, who helped me with the final production of this book in its final form.

Chapter One

PAIN IN PERSPECTIVE

Joyce's headaches began when she was a teenager and grew worse as she moved into her twenties. She married, had two children, and found a responsible but demanding job. Her life seemed to be going well, but the headaches continued. She found herself going from doctor to doctor and trying a variety of medications—all to no avail. At first, her husband was supportive and took over the family responsibilities whenever she was bedridden with a headache, but eventually he grew frustrated. He started staying away from home. The children began to have problems in school. She finally took a leave of absence from her job because she was missing so many days anyway. She knew she needed help desperately, but she had nowhere to turn.

Sam was a thirty-eight-year-old, burly, happy-go-lucky construction worker until he strained his back severely by lifting a heavy object at work. The pain was excruciating and forced him to stay home resting for many months. He took narcotic medications to ease his pain and hoped that his injuries would eventually heal themselves. When this did not happen, a surgeon suggested surgery and Sam agreed—anything to relieve the relentless pain he was suffering. The pain eased somewhat after the surgery, but it didn't go away. He became very upset with his doctor when the surgery "did not prove to be 100 percent successful." Another doctor prescribed different pain-relief medications. Initially they were helpful, but after a while the pain always came back. Sam was now a much different person than he had been before his accident. He was angry and depressed. He felt he was too young to resign himself to being an invalid for the rest of his life, but what other choice did he have?

Joyce and Sam are not alone. They are victims of chronic pain and are among the more than 30 percent of all Americans who regularly experience persistent, continuing pain. Their pain may be in their backs or joints, in their heads or stomachs, but wherever it is located, it affects their lives in dramatic and usually negative ways. At least one-third of these people are so completely disabled by their pain that they cannot carry out any type of normal daily activities.

Defining what the sufferers of chronic pain feel is very difficult. Each person experiences pain in a different way. In the next chapter, the differences between chronic pain and acute pain are explained more fully. But for the purpose of this chapter, chronic pain can be defined as long-term, persistent pain, which produces significant negative changes in the life of the person. There is usually no clear treatment to cure chronic pain. Acute pain, on the other hand, is of short-term duration and related to a specific event—such as surgery or an accident—from which the patient recovers completely.

Whether pain is chronic or acute, it is a complex experience that involves many intricate physical and emotional interactions. Our anxieties and beliefs about pain have a major impact on how it affects us, but one thing is certain—chronic pain is very real and extremely frustrating to those who suffer from it. As with Joyce and Sam, chronic pain involves every part of a person's life and unless it is handled effectively it can turn productive, positive people into miserable individuals with no hope for any happiness in their lives.

Chronic pain affects millions

The Nuprin Report published in 1985 reports on a survey by Louis Harris and Associates which emphasizes the prevalence and dramatic impact of pain on Americans. These results highlight the enormity of the problem for individuals, families, and society in general. Chronic pain is not just a problem for the sufferer. It is a problem for all of us.

For many Americans pain is only an occasional problem, but for countless others, pain has become a pervasive force in their lives. The Nuprin Report says that over 20 million adults reported suffering from chronic pain more than 100 days in 1984. These people reported pain from a variety of sources, including headaches, backaches, muscle pain, joint pain, and stomach pain.

One hundred days is a lot of time. These figures represent millions of Americans who are experiencing pain during a substantial part of their daily lives. Some of these people report continuous, intense pain. Their pain affects more than their own individual quality of life. It affects everyone around them.

Who suffers from chronic pain?

American families are intensely affected when a family member experiences chronic pain. The focus of the sufferer's life becomes his or her pain. Children and spouses are frequently neglected as the pain sufferer relentlessly pursues relief, or perhaps gives up, and retreats into a fog of hopelessness and depression. This book is addressed to family members as well as to pain victims. Family members sometimes are as much a part of the problem of chronic pain as the pain itself, because they unintentionally may be encouraging the sufferer to become dependent by taking over responsibilities and sympathizing to an unnecessary degree. Family members need to be part of the solution to the chronic pain problem.

American business suffers because of the loss in the work force. According to the Nuprin Report, Americans lose about 550 million workdays each year as a result of pain. The National Institute of Health estimates that the economic impact of pain on our economy (measured in terms of direct medical costs, lost income, lost productivity, compensation payments, and legal charges) comes to over $50 billion a year. These figures point to overwhelming losses in quality of life for many Americans and in production for our country's economy.

The Nuprin Report indicates that pain can affect any group of people when it comes to sex, age, race, or income, though there are certain groups that are more likely to suffer specific kinds of pain. People of all ages experience pain, but young people are more likely to experience pain in the form of headaches, backaches, muscle aches, stomachaches, menstrual pain, and dental pain. The incidence of joint pain increases sharply with age. Women are somewhat more likely to experience pain than men, especially when it comes to headaches. White Americans experience more pain than blacks or Hispanics, but there seems to be no dramatic difference between the prevalence of pain in different income groups.

The survey did indicate a strong familial and cultural link when it comes to pain. If your parents suffered from severe pain at some point in their lives, then it is more likely that you will suffer pain too. This characteristic seems more related to how one is raised as a child regarding reaction to pain, rather than to genetic or cultural heritage. Lifestyle also seems to have an impact on the likelihood of suffering from chronic pain. Generally, people who lead healthy lives suffer less from pain. If you exercise regularly, don't smoke and drink very little alcohol, you may not experience as much pain as a person who leads a less healthy life. Another interesting fact is that people who spend many hours watching television suffer more from headaches, backaches, and joint pains than people who don't.

These survey results and statistics may indicate the pervasiveness of pain, but they don't have much effect on you, the person in pain, except to say "you are not alone." For many sufferers, pain relief is the elusive pot of gold at the end of the rainbow—constantly pursued, but rarely attained. Pain sufferers may find themselves going around in a self-perpetuating circle of new medications and doctors, new therapies and miracle cures. They are frequently haunted by the public and sometimes private suspicion that their pain is "all in the head." Not infrequently, the pain sufferer questions his own sanity. He may ask himself, "Could I be imagining this pain? If so, why can't I imagine it away?"

Sufferers of chronic pain almost always are victims of their own low self-esteem. It is difficult to feel good about yourself when you are unable to assume your normal roles in life. When the homemaker cannot clean the house or take care of the children, when the truck driver cannot drive a truck, their feelings about themselves suffer. Reestablishing positive self-esteem is one of the first steps toward dealing with pain. It is also one of the hardest to achieve because chronic pain has resulted in a downward spiral away from productiveness in life and toward withdrawal and isolation.

Why this book?

This book has been written to address this pervasive problem. It is aimed at pain sufferers and their families. Its goal is not total release from pain, because that may be an impossible objective, but it aims instead to help the sufferer of chronic pain attain a satisfying quality of life and become once again a productive, contributing member of his or her family and society. You don't have to read every chapter of this book in order; you may pick and choose the chapters which will help you the most. Whatever parts of the book you read, you will find empathy and an understanding of the seriousness of your problem. First and foremost, this book acknowledges the reality of a person's pain. If you feel pain, *it is real* and must be managed as a real problem which needs to be solved. The specific goals in the treatment of patients with chronic persistent pain are as follows:

1. To return to your usual role in daily life

Sufferers of chronic pain usually have given up the regular patterns of their daily lives. They may not go to work or assume normal family responsibilities. They have frequently given up contributing to their families and communities. Family members and friends have assumed responsibilities for them and they are finding themselves out of touch with real living. Perhaps they do not drive or go to the grocery store as they used to. They don't play ball with their children or go to church on Sunday. They have retreated into their own gray world of continuing pain and are establishing a negative daily pattern of retreat and isolation. The goal is to establish their roles again— once again to become an active, contributing family member—once again to become an effective worker and member of the community—to get up in the morning with goals and objectives. This may mean some changes in roles or going back to a different job, but the point is to be a productive person again.

2. To eliminate or decrease pain-induced behaviors

The chronic pain sufferer develops patterns of behavior which characterize that person's pain. It may be grimacing when moving. It may be constant complaining. It may be limping while walking. It may be worrying about and anticipating pain before it even occurs. Whatever the behavior is, its elimination will be a positive step toward living a full life. By imitating the positive behaviors of those who are free of pain, an individual's pain will lessen and the mind will focus on more productive endeavors.

3. To learn skills to cope with pain

Eliminating pain completely is not always a realistic goal, but certain skills can be learned to help people live with pain more comfortably and improve your ability to function. The first step toward learning these skills may be to learn more about pain and how it develops. Knowing not only what is wrong with them, but also what is right with them is a major step in control of pain. Each individual needs to find his or her own method for best handling pain. It may be meditation or relaxation techniques. It may be exercising or visual imaging. It may be appropriate medications. It may be learning how to develop the positive frame of mind that allows one to accept some pain and motivates a person to go on living productively anyway. It may be learning to pace activities so that they are achievable and not stressful. *This book is about learning the techniques not only to live with pain but to function despite it.*

4. To increase physical activity

Persistent pain has a way of making us stop moving—even when movement may be just what we need to rehabilitate our joints and muscles and to distract us from our pain. Whether it's walking or climbing stairs, swimming or playing golf, shopping or bicycling, the goal is *to move*. You may start slowly and then gradually build up the length of time you are active. It may hurt at first, but activity usually will help your pain decrease in the long run. Individuals learn the difference between "hurting," or a personal sense of discomfort, versus "harm," which could damage the body.

5. To increase independence

Sufferers of chronic pain frequently become almost totally dependent on family members to get them through their lives. They may not drive a car or walk to the post office. They are supported both financially and physically by others. They become completely dependent, depressed individuals who have lost control of their own behaviors and decisions. The goal is to get them back on their feet as functioning human beings who can take care of their own needs and be responsible for their own happiness.

6. To eliminate or decrease the use of dependence-producing (and nonessential) medications

For many pain sufferers, narcotic medications provide their only relief. After a while, the sufferer needs more and more medicine which gives less and less relief. Medications create their own cycle of side effects which actually may intensify the problem of living with pain. These medications may be very effective in handling temporary or acute pain, but a tolerance usually develops when they are used for a long period of time. They may make the mind foggy and produce other undesirable conditions such as constipation, drowsiness, nausea, or depression.

Medications may dull a person's pain temporarily, but ultimately they will also dull a person's capacity for living life to the fullest. For most sufferers of chronic pain, completely eliminating narcotic drugs is a positive step which opens the door to dealing with the problem of pain rather than covering up the symptoms temporarily. Eventually, you may occasionally use appropriate medications, but first you must eliminate all narcotics.

Chronic pain treatment—HOPE

Achieving these goals is especially important because of the failure of traditional approaches in achieving long-term pain relief. Doctors tend to find chronic pain a terrible problem because they do not know how to manage it. They have learned to manage acute or temporary pain, but pain that persists is a completely different condition. Patients come to doctors expecting miracle cures and when these cures are not delivered, patients become angry. Frequently, surgery is offered as an alternative, but it rarely eliminates chronic pain totally and is likely to create other problems. Surgery may alleviate one source of pain, but may replace it with another. Prescription analgesics can cause many of the problems mentioned earlier and are a symptomatic treatment which can stand in the way of addressing the pain itself. Mental health professionals, including psychiatrists, may help you start to confront the problem of chronic pain, but some of them are inexperienced in the complex problems of the chronic pain sufferer. They formulate their approaches according to other mental health conditions, which are not the same as those of patients with chronic pain.

On a positive note, the individual who suffers from chronic pain has more reason to hope now than ever before. Modern technology is beginning to offer more alternatives, and research is starting to reveal more about the complex process of pain and pain relief. A growing number of support groups and pain rehabilitation programs throughout the country promise a successful approach for many sufferers. Combined with an optimistic mental attitude, this all points toward your ability to live with pain and still enjoy life. Success stories similar to the one described below are repeated again and again. *Pain IS a four-letter word you can live with.*

Martha was only thirty years old when she first started to feel the symptoms of arthritis. Over the next two years, her pain had become almost debilitating. Her condition was diagnosed as fibromyalgia, and not as an active arthritis disorder. But due to pain, she gave up her weekly golf game and started socializing with her friends less and began complaining more. Once an extremely active person, she began taking a variety of medications for pain relief and spent many drowsy days at home in front of the television. It took the insistence of her husband to get her to participate reluctantly in a pain rehabilitation program at a local hospital. There she shared her frustrations with others suffering chronic pain. She learned techniques to deal with her pain and realized that she was responsible for her own happiness. Today at the age of thirty-seven, her pain is not gone but it bothers her much less. Hours and sometimes even days go by when she is

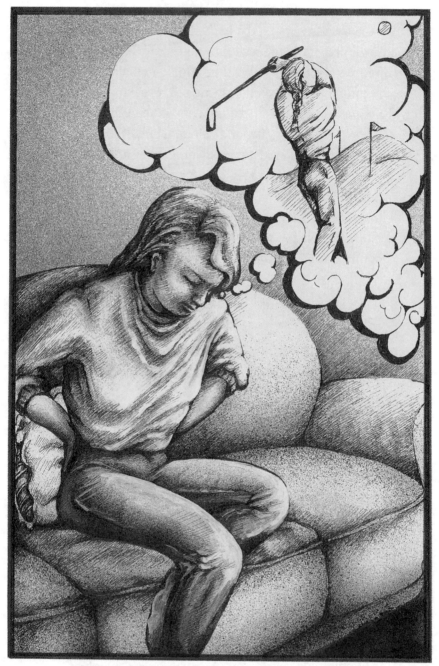

Figure 1: The chronic pain dilemma—HOPE

hardly aware of pain. She has decreased her pain relieving medications drastically, and uses them very appropriately now. She has resumed her golfing, keeps a regular bridge date with her friends, and is back in the swing of life again. She has learned not only to live with her pain but to live a life that is full and satisfying. She is in control of her pain and her life.

KEY POINTS TO REMEMBER

Chronic pain is long-term and persistent. Acute pain is short-term and related to a specific event—such as surgery or an injury—from which the patient recovers.

According to the Nuprin Report (1985), Americans lose 550 million workdays each year due to pain. The National Institute of Health estimates the economic cost of pain to be in the range of over $50 billion annually.

By and large, people who lead healthy lives suffer less from pain. A healthy lifestyle includes healthy eating habits, an exercise schedule, and the effective management of stress.

Chronic pain can rarely be completely cured. Neither surgery nor medications can relieve most chronic pain. The primary steps in controlling pain involve a positive emotional attitude, a healthy lifestyle, and learning to be responsible for yourself.

Chapter Two

PAIN: A FOUR-LETTER WORD THAT'S HARD TO DEFINE

John grew up in a family where every little sign of illness or discomfort was taken seriously. Whenever he had a slightly runny nose or a cough, his mother allowed him to stay home from school and comforted him with hot chicken broth and lots of loving attention. His parents and other relatives had various minor ailments which were the main discussion topics at many family gatherings. When John started to have chronic back pain, he moved easily into his family's pattern of dealing with

15

discomfort. He stayed home from work and tried to take it easy. When the pain worsened, he became frustrated and angry, but he also remembered his parents' continuous suffering and assumed there was little he could do.

Tim, on the other hand, grew up in a family that didn't seem to have time to be sick. His parents owned their own retail outlet and worked most weekends and evenings, no matter how they felt. He, too, was expected to carry his fair share of family responsibilities without complaint. He knew better than to shirk work because of a bad cold or headache. It was only when his mother was close to death that he learned she had worked steadily and uncomplainingly over the years despite the relentless progression of arthritis. When Tim was injured severely in an automobile accident, his recovery was termed miraculous by his physicians. Despite continuing leg pain, he was back at work in four weeks and the only reminder of the accident seemed to be a barely perceptible limp. Six months after his accident, he was promoted to a managerial position, in great part, according to his boss, because of his "dedication to work despite all obstacles."

Pain: an individual experience

These two examples may seem extreme, but they do reflect how individual differences in reacting to pain are deeply ingrained within us. Pain should not be ignored as it was in Tim's family, especially if it is acute and recurring, since it may be a symptom of something wrong; however, John allowed his pain to fall right into his family patterns and consequently it immobilized him. While Tim seemed to use his accident as an opportunity to move ahead in his job, John used his pain to retreat from challenge and everyday life. There is no doubt that sensitivity to pain seems to run in families and sometimes in particular cultures or societies. Our family histories and ethnic or cultural heritage play a significant role in how we perceive pain and cope with it when it strikes us.

Our society has some stereotyped concepts of how various ethnic groups experience pain. For instance, Germans are felt to be stoic and unfeeling when it comes to pain while Italians are perceived as emotional and prone to experiencing great pain. These perceptions do not always hold true. Germans can hurt just as much as Italians hurt; however, studies have shown that there are differences in how families from different ethnic backgrounds raise their children to experience pain. Ethnic or cultural groups seem to establish patterns in the ways they face illness or pain. The resulting differences, then, are based more on the environment in which a child is raised than on innate genetic differences. Children raised in families like John's seem to be more affected by pain than children raised in families like Tim's, whatever their nationality.

Our individual personalities and emotional and physical makeup also have a major impact on how we experience pain, as does the timing of a painful experience. If we are going through a particularly stressful time in our lives, then we may experience pain more intensely than if our lives are fairly stable. There is no doubt that there is a close relationship between the mind and the body in the pain experience.

Trying to define pain

Defining pain and measuring it objectively, then, becomes almost impossible because pain is such a personal experience and is influenced by so many factors. We can go so far as to say that *pain is a subjective sensation of distress, agony, or discomfort caused by a complex interaction of various stimuli with the mind.* Pain frequently is associated with tissue, bone, or organ damage and it is the most common symptom that brings a patient to the physician.

The International Association for the Study of Pain (IASP) describes pain as "An unpleasant sensory or emotional experience that is associated with tissue damage or described in terms of such, or both." The bottom line for most of us, however, is that pain hurts!

There is no doubt that the word *pain* suggests an unpleasant or negative experience. The word itself is derived from both the Sanskrit word *pu* meaning sacrifice and the Latin word *poena* meaning punishment. The word is often used to describe unpleasant non-physical experiences. When speaking of a boring, unfriendly acquaintance, we may say, "He is a pain," or when talking about a tedious job we may say, "It's a pain to get up in the morning and go to work."

Acute pain: a necessity and a help

This negative association with pain is not really appropriate because pain is actually a necessity. It functions to our benefit most of the time. Pain is a warning signalling that something is wrong. Pain tells us when we have broken a bone or sprained an ankle, when we have an infected ear, appendicitis, or serious indigestion. Pain may warn us of a heart attack taking place or a cancer developing inside of us. We would become very ill or perhaps even die if we did not have pain to tell us something is wrong. This kind of warning signal pain is termed *acute pain*. It is a meaningful and useful sensation which signals a physical condition needing attention. Fortunately, acute pain is also usually short-term. It goes away when the physical condition is adequately evaluated and treated.

Chronic pain: the problem

This book, however, is about *chronic pain*—pain that is not necessarily connected with an identifiable physical condition, pain for which there is no obvious treatment, and pain which is long-term, lasting well beyond the expected healing period for the initial condition. A key part of the definition of chronic pain is its significant negative impact on a person's life, leading to major lifestyle changes such as loss of employment, less satisfying relationships with friends and family, decreased activity and a range of psychological changes, including depression, drug abuse, and loss of self-confidence.

The causes of chronic pain can elude even the most experienced physicians. Pain may last for many years after damaged tissues have healed and nerves have regenerated. The classic example is the pain a person may feel in a limb which actually has been amputated. The patient may say, "My foot hurts," when he has no foot. This phantom pain seems to have no clear cause, yet it is very real to the person experiencing it.

On the other hand, it is possible to experience an injury with no pain. Your skin may be badly burned by the sun, but you don't feel any pain until several hours after the burn occurs, or you fall down and hit your knee but don't realize that you have been cut until you see blood coming through your clothing. Just like injury or disease is not always associated with pain, it is important to realize pain can occur without injury or disease always being identified.

Chronic pain may be located almost anywhere in the body—the back, head, neck, joints, stomach, muscles, or nerves. It can have a variety of initial causes from injuries, disc herniations, arthritis, migraine headaches, dental problems, ulcers, or whiplash injuries. Pain caused by a cancer, though it has some of the characteristics of both acute and chronic pain, in most situations requires different treatment because of its cause and possible outcome. However, some of the information described in this book may be of some benefit to cancer patients and their families.

Legal and healthcare systems affect the pain experience

Another reality is that a person's involvement in the legal or healthcare systems may have an impact on pain. Studies have shown that some individuals who are involved in litigation concerning injuries related to pain experience little pain relief until the case is settled. The healthcare system, too, has been known to aggravate pain. When an individual suffering chronic pain has gone from doctor to doctor, undergone a number of surgeries, tried a range of powerful medications—all to no avail—

that person frequently feels that his pain is hopeless and that he is a victim of just the system he was sure could provide relief.

The first step in handling pain may be to recognize that chronic, not acute, pain is the culprit to be managed. Because of its complexity and its impact on so many facets of our lives, chronic pain needs to be managed differently from acute pain. The chart at the end of this chapter will help you decide whether the pain you are suffering can be classified as chronic pain.

If you are suffering from chronic pain, you may be able to identify with the words of New England poet Emily Dickinson:

"*Pain—has an Element of Blank —*
It cannot recollect
When it begun—or if there were
A time when it was not."

Chronic pain check list:

Answer the following questions for yourself or for a family member. The more questions to which you answer *yes*, the more likely it is that you are experiencing chronic pain.

Y N

☐ ☐ Has your pain lasted longer than is usually the case with the physical condition you experienced?

☐ ☐ Has your pain lasted longer than six months?

☐ ☐ Has your pain affected your ability to go to work or to function effectively at your job?

☐ ☐ Have you visited different doctors or clinics looking for relief from your pain?

Y N

☐ ☐ Have you tried more than one unsuccessful approach to treating your pain—such as multiple medications or surgeries?

☐ ☐ Do you find yourself feeling any of the following:
  — anger
  — frustration
  — loss of self-confidence
  — depression
  — hopelessness
  — irritability

☐ ☐ Do you find yourself turning to alcohol or drugs for temporary relief?

☐ ☐ Do you find yourself becoming more and more dependent on prescribed medications, particularly narcotics?

☐ ☐ Are you less active than you used to be? Do you exercise less? Have you given up a number of activities that you used to enjoy?

☐ ☐ Does the focus of your life seem to be your pain? Do you find it hard to think about or discuss other topics?

☐ ☐ Is your sleep disturbed or interrupted several times? Do you feel tired and not rested?

☐ ☐ Have your work or social activities been affected due to pain?

What pain is and is not

Pain Is	Pain Is Not
Real	Imaginary
Complex	Simple
Different for everyone	The same for everyone
Of varying degrees	Measurable
What hurts!	

KEY POINTS TO REMEMBER

Pain prompts different people to react differently. Our family histories and ethnic or cultural heritage play a significant role in how we perceive pain and cope with it when it strikes.

It is hard to define the concept of pain in a few words. However, pain can be described as a subjective unpleasant sensation of distress, agony, or discomfort caused by a complex interaction of various stimuli with the mind.

While the experience of pain is negative, acute pain is self-limiting. It is helpful to both the person with the pain and the caring physician in that it warns that something is wrong, and is resolved after the problem is treated.

Chronic pain becomes persistent, lasting beyond the usual healing period, and has no identifiable treatment to cure it.

The distinguishing feature of *chronic pain* is its significant negative impact on a person's life, leading to major lifestyle changes. Chronic pain must be handled very differently from acute pain.

Chapter Three

HOW PAIN WORKS

Trudy had always been an active, involved person, but as she grew older she started experiencing sporadic aches and pains in her back. Her doctor said she had mild arthritis and prescribed some medications, but that didn't seem to help. Finally, about the time she turned sixty-five, the pain became more intense and more continuous. She went from doctor to doctor and still could not uncover the cause of all her pain. Several times, doctors implied that it might be "all in her head," which made her very angry because she knew her pain was real and she had never been a complaining person. Even her friends and family members shook their heads at her inability to get on with life. As her anger and frustration increased, so did her pain. One morning she woke up and thought, "Today it hurts too much to even get out of bed and no one can help me. No one else I know has ever felt this way for no reason. There is no answer to this pain." She had never felt so depressed or hopeless in her whole life.

How pain works

Understanding how pain works is a key step in relieving or controlling it. If Trudy had been given an explanation for her disabling pain—especially an explanation tied in with pain management techniques, she probably would have more control over her pain. Sometimes just knowing that it is not unusual to undergo unaccountable pain can help a person feel she is not alone in her struggle and give her the motivation to keep trying. If a physician can identify a cause or explain how a person's pain reflects an established theory about pain, then a treatment plan can be initiated. The problem arises when pain remains an inexplicable and mysterious condition.

Since pain is such a universal experience, scientists have been trying to explain it for centuries. Various theories have been developed to explain the existence of pain and the different approaches to managing it. Each of the major theories outlined in this chapter has something to teach us about why we feel pain and how we can start to control it. Keep in mind, however, that pain is hard to define, difficult to measure, and not always possible to describe precisely. No one theory can provide the answer to the problem of pain, but theories can help us start to understand what is going on in our bodies. Understanding and knowledge are the first steps toward acceptance and control.

The Bell theory

Over 350 years ago, the specificity theory (doorbell theory) of pain was first introduced. This theory proposes that a specific pain system carries messages from pain receptors in the skin to a pain center in the brain. Thus, the pain system was conceived as a direct channel linking nerves from the skin and other tissues to the brain. This theory has been compared to the ringing mechanism of a doorbell. When the bell rings, it is usually due to someone pushing the button by the door. In response to this ringing, you reach for the door. Likewise, when you touch a hot stove or bang your finger with a hammer, your immediate response is to feel pain, due to the direct connection between the finger and brain through nerves. Injury to tissues leads to release of chemicals, such as Bradykinin, Prostaglandin, Histamine, and Substance P (a pain-producing substance). These initiate the pain process (Nocioception—see page 36) by stimulating the nerve endings (the doorbell). The nerves then carry the message to the brain, where it is perceived as pain (the bell rings). Medications such as aspirin work by blocking the release of these chemicals (Chapter 5). Your reaction to the pain is much like answering the doorbell or telephone when you hear a ring. The bell theory is illustrated in Figure 2.

The bell theory is a simple explanation of some of the characteristics of pain but not all of them. You need to understand how this system works and how it doesn't work. There are receptors that carry temperature or pressure messages with a certain degree of intensity, and after these sensations reach the spinal cord, they are changed and modified to reach the brain. If the brain

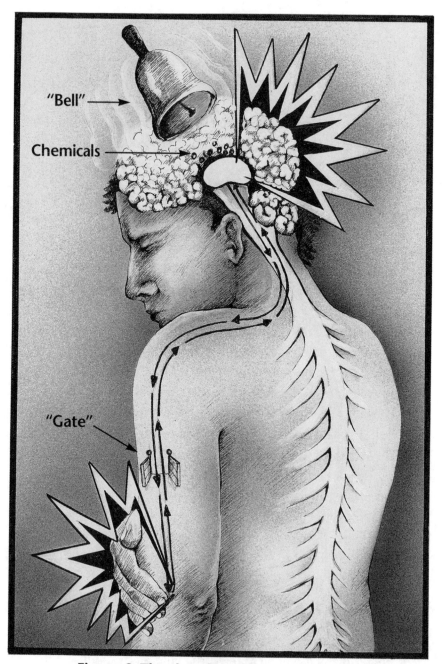

Figure 2: The theories of how pain works

perceives this as pain, then the appropriate sensation and related emotions occur.

The bell theory of pain explains why pain may be felt even though nothing specific can be found on tests—just as a faulty doorbell may ring and no one may be at the door. The bell continues to ring and we keep opening doors—to no avail. The message here is to stop opening the door. Stop undergoing numerous, unnecessary tests. Stop expecting the healthcare system to do things that won't work and may even aggravate the problem. An effective pain management program can help you learn ways to ignore the ringing bells. If you do something else other than opening the door, you will not be letting pain in.

While we may feel pain when there is no apparent injury, we also may suffer injuries and yet not feel the pain. Have you ever cut yourself, drawing blood without pain, or suddenly noticed a bruise on your arm or leg without remembering the pain that should have accompanied the injury that produced the bruise? This concept of the unanswered signal is also part of the bell theory. What happens if you don't hear the bell ring? Obviously, you don't answer it; however, someone may be trying very hard to reach you and be unable to make the connection. Perhaps you are out in the yard and too far away from the phone. Or maybe other sounds such as a loud TV program are drowning out the ring. Perhaps you just weren't paying attention, or the doorbell system is faulty. Whatever the reason, the connection is not made. The same thing happens sometimes with our pain pathways. For example, soldiers in battle sometimes experience significant injuries without reporting feeling the pain associated with these wounds.

Another part of the bell theory is the concept that the nerve pathways can be interrupted. For example, when a local anesthetic such as novocaine is used by dentists, nerves are blocked so that the patient doesn't feel pain when cavities are filled or teeth are pulled. Anesthesiologists use spinal blocks or epidural blocks during surgery so the patient may remain awake but still not feel pain.

The bell theory doesn't work when we look at certain kinds of patients. For instance, we all know that a person who has had a limb amputated may still feel pain in that limb. This phantom pain exists even though the direct channel between the missing limb and the brain has obviously been severed. Explanations for this phenomenon are that the nerve ending in the amputated stump may be irritated or that the brain continues to remember the pain even though its cause is gone. Similarly, patients who are paralyzed sometimes may feel pain in that portion of the body where they otherwise have no sensation.

In attempting to relieve pain, surgeons throughout the last century have tried to interrupt the system which carries the sensation of pain by surgically cutting nerves in the limbs or spinal cord; this approach, however, does not always abolish pain. Some patients experience only temporary pain relief, and some find that their pain grows worse, both in severity and in the affected area of the body. These techniques are still used, but only rarely and in patients with severe uncontrollable pain due to advanced cancer.

Despite its shortcomings, the bell theory describes a good warning system which is usually very helpful to the patient and physician in understanding some sources of pain and setting up a treatment plan. It is just as important to keep in mind the fact that the bell may not ring even though an injury has occurred, and that at other times, the bell may ring continuously though there appears to be no injury or damage. This was the case with Trudy whose bell kept ringing but no cause or answer emerged. When this happens, patients and physicians understandably become very frustrated because this kind of pain is so difficult to understand and treat.

When pain persists, seemingly without cause or reason, patients turn first to their physicians for immediate solutions. When these solutions aren't forthcoming, the healthcare system and physicians, in particular, often are blamed. Doctors are perplexed because there appears to be no obvious source of the pain, making the condition very difficult to treat and to explain to their patients.

Gate control theory

Two scientists named Melzack and Wall introduced the gate control theory in 1965. Though this is a complex theory involving the relationship of sensory nerves in perceiving pain, the basic message is, "If you rub it, pain may be decreased." This theory says that there is a gate-like mechanism in the spinal cord which determines whether pain is perceived or not. Nerve impulses from fibers outside the brain are modified by the gate as they enter the spinal cord. Large fiber activity brings in non-painful types of sensation and small fiber activity brings in painful sensations. Large fibers can block, change, or decrease the information brought in by the small fibers, which are carrying the pain messages (Figure 3).

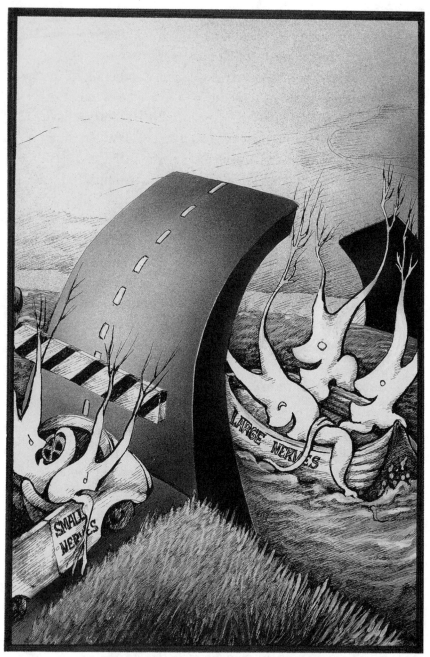

Figure 3: The gate theory of pain

The gate is also influenced by nerve impulses which come from the brain. In this way, negative emotions, such as anger, frustration, anxiety, and depression can open the gate while relaxation and other pain management techniques (see Chapter 5) can decrease the pain by closing the gate.

Stimuli such as rubbing or heat prompts the large nerve fibers to modify or stop the painful impulse. Or, to use a scientific approach, the skin could be stimulated using an electrical current just intensely enough to affect the large fibers but not the small pain fibers. If, on the other hand, you suffer a puncture wound or severe blow which arouses the small nerve fibers, the gate opens and pain comes charging in.

Most of us can identify with the relief of pain which can accompany massaging or rubbing a sore area of the body. When our feet ache, we rub them, and when our backs ache, we long for a massage. Rubbing doesn't always work, but when it does, the gate theory is reinforced. Pain treatment based on the gate theory involves stimulating those fibers which close rather than open the gate.

When the gate theory was first proposed, the reaction was controversial. After all, it challenged the long-accepted bell theory which was simpler and easier to understand; however, the test of time has shown the gate control theory to be an effective explanation for many pain problems. It has helped generate a variety of successful pain management techniques. Though techniques such as massage, stretching exercises, heat application, and electrical stimulations have been known for a long time to relieve pain, the gate theory provides an explanation of why they work. In chronic pain management, movement is also very important, and may help by closing the gate.

The Chemical theory

The chemical theory of pain involves the release of *endorphins*, *enkephalins*, and other chemicals produced in the body. Just as prescribed analgesics may help us control pain, this theory says that there are pain-suppressing chemicals in the brain which need to be released to affect pain. The theory is that endorphins, chemicals that are released from brain cells, act like morphine and inhibit pain through pathways between the brain and spinal cord. Endorphins also might be released by painful procedures and vigorous exercises. Obviously, a treatment plan which successfully activates natural pain-suppressing chemicals is more desirable than an approach which uses narcotic pain relievers with their undesirable side effects. Similarly, use of antidepressant medications for treating pain is more common now, as it has been shown that these increase certain chemicals. The neurotransmitters such as *Norepinephrine* and *Serotonin* are increased in the brain with antidepressants such as *Amitryptyline* (Elavil®). Such medications are especially useful in patients with chronic pain (see Chapter 5).

Theories abound about what causes pain and how to treat it because scientists have searched long and hard for answers to this perplexing problem. However, the explanation of these three theories should help you reach a basic concept of what is going on in your body when you feel pain and also of how complex it is to treat pain. It is important to remember that doctors use these theories to develop treatments to help you learn how to manage and live with your pain.

Hypersensitivity to pain

Another point to keep in mind is that the body has a tendency to develop a hypersensitivity to pain after nerve injury has occurred, further intensifying the pain a person experiences. If you've ever had a frostbitten foot or sunburn, you know that those areas are more painful to touch than other parts of your body which have never been damaged. When you stub your toe or sunburn your back these areas remain very painful to touch for some time after the injury.

This sensitivity after tissue damage is due to the release of chemicals which, in turn, make the skin more sensitive to pain. Aspirin and other anti-inflammatory drugs reduce pain by preventing release of some of these chemicals.

However, in certain conditions, such as with some patients after shingles, severe pain develops in the shingles area. This is called *Post-herpetic Neuralgia*. After minor injuries, patients sometimes develop severe hypersensitivity, pain, and coldness (Reflex Sympathetic Dystrophy Syndrome). These are some examples of chronic pain, where the nerves have "gone crazy" and caused hypersensitivity.

This is a very simplified explanation of the theories that deal with what causes pain. (If you are interested in more detailed explanations, see the bibliography at the back of this book.) People like Trudy need to know that many factors are involved in the persistence of chronic pain.

Important terms to remember

It is also important here to recognize some important terms. John Loeser, M.D., from the University of Washington in Seattle, proposed a new way of viewing pain. This includes:

a) Nocioception—*the chemical, thermal, or mechanical energy which irritates the nerves and initiates the "doorbell" mechanism.*

b) Pain—*the sensation when nocioception is perceived by the brain (the bell rings).*

c) Suffering—*the emotional response triggered by pain and nocioception, including fear and anxiety.*

d) Pain behaviors—*things people say and do which may indicate that they are in pain, including sleeping, complaining, taking medications, missing work, and becoming dependent on family and the health care system. There may be factors other than pain and nocioception that trigger pain behaviors as well.*

Dr. Wilbert Fordyce, a psychologist from the University of Washington, has expanded on this proposal. He has clearly shown that pain behaviors can be modified by changing those factors that are perceived as positive reinforcers of those behaviors. Rewarding "well behaviors" with attention and ignoring "pain behaviors" are major steps in chronic pain management (see Chapter 5).

Cognitive factors—how the brain understands the meaning of pain also plays a major role in labeling pain and suffering. Anticipation of pain and fear are cognitive factors that affect perception and reaction to pain. Patients can be taught the difference between *hurt* and *harm*. Dr. Fordyce has emphasized that pain does not necessarily mean that healing has not occurred, a residual injury is present, or further harm is going to take place. Patients can be taught "to make it better, use it." He emphasizes that "people who have something better to do don't suffer as much."

A specialist in managing pain might say to her, "Trudy, your pain is real but hard to explain. There are intricate wiring systems and chemical combinations in your body that are somehow interacting to generate this pain. Because of the complexity of your pain, we may not be able to eliminate it completely, but we can help you learn to live with it. There are many pain management techniques which have been developed out of extensive research into the causes of pain. Many other people have gone through the same kind of experience and they have learned ways to control their pain. You can learn to have this kind of control too." That's what this book is all about.

Trudy's story has a happy ending. Just as she was giving up, a good friend persuaded her to visit a pain clinic at a local hospital. Through the understanding and expertise of a team of specialists, she learned ways in which she could have some control over her pain. She learned relaxation techniques and practiced focusing her attention on ideas and objects other than her pain. As her mood changed from anger to acceptance, she was enabling the "gate" to close. She learned to rub the area that hurt, stimulating the large fibers which also helped close the gate. She started a routine of regular walking every day, very slowly at first and then somewhat faster. She is now to the point where the intensity of her pain is rarely disabling, though it still exists. She can go for many hours without even thinking about it. Her life is almost normal again and her attitude is positive and optimistic.

KEY POINTS TO REMEMBER

Understanding pain and how it works is a key step in relieving or controlling it. Scientists have developed various theories to explain pain, but no one theory is capable of providing a complete solution to explain each person's pain.

The BELL theory of pain says it is possible to control chronic pain by ignoring pain signals, diverting your attention, or simply drowning it out with distracting activities (Figure 2, page 28).

Pain treatment based on the GATE control theory involves stimulating certain fibers that close the gate-like mechanism in the spinal cord which determines the perception of pain. Thus, techniques such as rubbing, applying heat or an electric current can "close" the gate to pain (Figure 3, page 32).

The CHEM theory of pain explains how pain can be controlled by stimulating the release of natural pain suppressing chemicals in the brain through methods such as exercise and certain antidepressant medications.

Chapter Four

CHRONIC BENIGN
PAIN SYNDROME:
WHAT IS IT?

Joe is a forty-three-year-old worker who has had continuing back pain after a work-related injury. After three months of rest and medications, the pain does not go away: A CAT scan (a special x-ray to look for a disc problem) is done. This reveals a large bulging disc and a nerve test indicates irritated nerves. His doctor treats this condition with cortisone injections and advises bed rest. This approach provides only temporary relief and the pain returns. *After surgery is performed on the disc, Joe experiences a dramatic relief of his symptoms; however, within two months the pain is back and seems even worse. Another CAT scan reveals scar tissue and the possibility that the disc is bulging again. Surgery is repeated but instead of decreasing, the pain increases.*

Joe's frustration mounts and he becomes increasingly angry at his physicians who cannot seem to find a solution to his problems and his employer who has not found a position for him with fewer physical demands. Joe's lack of employment is starting to have an economic impact on his family, increasing his distress and the pressure he feels to recover. He starts increasing his narcotic medications to help get him through the day. Sometimes he combines prescription medicines with alcohol to produce a numbing effect which temporarily helps him forget all his worries. However, his sleep is disturbed and he rarely sleeps more than two hours at a stretch. Joe can no longer find pleasure in life as he did in the past. He doesn't bowl or golf with his friends. His wife and children respond to his every request for help because they so desperately want him to be happy again. He slouches in front of the TV and worries about his family, his job, his life . . . .

J oe has Chronic Benign Pain Syndrome, usually called CBPS (Figure 4). He has many of the typical characteristics of the person so disabled by chronic pain that he is unable to function normally. The expected healing period after surgery has passed, and his doctor can

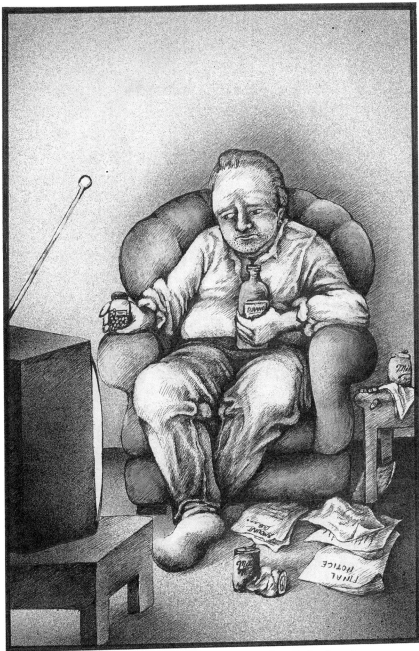

Figure 4: A patient with Chronic Benign Pain Syndrome

detect no active disease that can be improved with medical, physical, or surgical treatment. The usual therapies, including rest, numerous medications, cortisone shots, and physical therapy, have resulted in no noticeable improvement. Most importantly, his pain has had a devastating impact on every facet of his life—everything from his job to his social and family relationships has been affected negatively. Joe's only hope for ever leading a normal life begins with recognizing the symptoms of CBPS. (In this and subsequent chapters, chronic pain and CBPS are used interchangeably.)

The first step in learning to manage chronic pain is to understand what CBPS is and recognize it in yourself. The goal of this chapter is to guide you in that process—to help you understand your condition and see that your symptoms are not isolated but work together to create the frustrating and disabling condition that medical professionals refer to as CBPS. (The next chapter takes you beyond recognition of your condition to learn not only how to live with pain, but how to function despite it.)

What does *chronic* mean?

The word *chronic* means something that has lasted beyond a certain period of time. Six months is used in most medical circles as a landmark lapse of time to differentiate between acute and chronic pain. Most acute pain conditions seem to be resolved within three months, at the longest. But healthcare professionals dealing with patients with persistent pain emphasize that chronic does not only refer to a period of time but to a condition that does not have a clearly identifiable process which can be treated using medical or surgical approaches.

What does *benign* mean?

Benign implies a simple process in contrast to *malignant* which means a progressive, destructive process. Malignancy usually means cancer. Though benign and malignant pain have some of the same characteristics such as their relatively long-term persistence, they are treated differently because their cause and potential outcomes are very different. Consequently, malignant pain (pain related to cancer) is usually treated aggressively with pain-reducing drugs.

Because it is compared to malignant pain, benign pain is sometimes not considered very serious. But patients with CBPS have a very serious problem. Like Joe, their lives are totally disrupted and their ability to function normally is impaired.

What does *syndrome* mean?

Syndrome means a group of symptoms and signs—which in this case indicate the presence of CBPS. Symptoms are indicated by the patient's complaints—a headache, a backache, watery eyes, aching joints, a depressed feeling, and so on. Signs are what the physician sees by examining the patient or conducting tests—x-rays or lab tests, or any other electrical, chemical, physical or psychological testing.

Consequently, someone with CBPS has many of the symptoms and signs which are characteristic of this group. The characteristics which follow are all part of the syndrome, as are the specific signs of the syndrome which doctors may uncover during their examinations and testing. For instance, depression as reported by the patient may be a symptom of CBPS, while specific psychological tests provide objective signs of depression.

Do you have CBPS?

When you can acknowledge the symptoms of CBPS in yourself, then you can start to deal with your pain effectively. If you, or someone close to you, has CBPS it is likely that you have many of the following symptoms:

- Pain is the major focus of your life. You wake up with pain. You go to bed with pain. You think about your pain most of the day.

- You have suffered major losses from the life you used to lead. You may have lost your job, friendships or relationships that once were important to you, in addition to your capacity to find enjoyment in life.

- You are feeling depressed most of the time. You find yourself looking at life negatively and worrying about the future. There is a sense of hopelessness about almost everything you do.

- You are dependent on drugs or alcohol to find relief from your pain. It's hard to get through a day or even a few hours without turning to some substance—whether it is alcohol or prescribed or over the counter (OTC) medications or both.

- You find yourself depending on others to accomplish the tasks you used to perform with ease. You are dependent on others for life's necessities. Someone else shops, cooks, and earns a living. In a sense, you have reverted to a childlike state where you want to be cared for by others rather than taking any responsibility for yourself.

• You may find yourself depending on the medical profession and healthcare system to continue to provide care and answers to your pain problem. You are constantly turning to the health care (medical) system for the magical cure which always seems to elude you.

• You are worried about money. Your financial security is becoming shakier by the minute since you are no longer able to make a living.

• You have experienced a history of treatment failures. Physical therapy, a range of medications, surgeries—you've tried or at least considered them all and nothing seems to work.

• You go from doctor to doctor. Each one tells you much the same thing: your physical condition does not indicate that you should have as much pain or disability as you have. Because of this lack of medical explanation for your pain, you are told that a cure is unlikely.

• There are "external incentives," or reasons outside of the presence of your pain, which may be motivating you—on *either a conscious or subconscious level*—to avoid resuming a normal life. Financial compensation for your disability may depend on your pain continuing. You may even be involved in a lawsuit, the success of which is dependent on proof of your continuing pain and disability. You may be receiving attention from loved ones you would not get if you were not disabled.

• Your behavior and approach to living is characterized by withdrawal. You are a melancholy and bitter observer of life rather than a participant. Your approach is "I can't," rather than "I can try!"

These multiple symptoms are characteristic of chronic pain and not acute pain. Most patients seem able to deal with acute pain because it is a time-limited condition which serves a useful function. Patients who have had surgery, for instance, expect to experience pain and treat it effectively with narcotics. Patients with chronic pain may try the typical approaches for dealing with acute pain and become very discouraged when they don't work. For acute pain there is usually a cure. For chronic pain, there is frequently no cure.

In most pain rehabilitation programs, patients are advised not to look for a cure. As is explained further in Chapter 5 on managing CBPS, constantly looking for a cure is a symptom of CBPS. It is unrealistic and actually destructive to many patients. *The turning point for many patients comes with the realization that though no cure exists, there can be significant improvement and an opportunity to lead a full life again.*

CBPS is not just a medical issue. It also involves the social and psychological aspects of a person's life. Effective treatment demands an understanding of the relationships among all these aspects. The psychological characteristics are just as important to understand as the physical ones, and though there are some common symptoms, each person with chronic pain is different. Each person's symptoms, when combined with his or her individual personality and history, result in a condition and eventual treatment approach that will be unique to that person. The complexity of CBPS is reflected in the following case:

Susan is a sixty-four-year-old, recently-widowed woman who fell at home. She is diagnosed as having a fractured hip and undergoes a surgical hip replacement with the initial result of excellent relief of her pain. However, after several weeks, her pain recurs. Numerous x-rays and bone scans reveal no obvious medical reason for her pain. Medication provides little relief. Meanwhile, her life has changed drastically. Once an independent woman who ran her home beautifully and participated in many volunteer activities, she now finds herself forced to live with her children. Every three months she moves from one child's home to another. She talks about living independently again but says, in the same breath, that this is impossible because of her constant pain. In a pain rehabilitation program, it becomes clear that she is deriving a great deal of attention from her children due to her pain. Rather than just seeing her grandchildren on holidays, she is enjoying seeing them grow up on a day-to-day basis. Her children take her to social functions that she enjoys and otherwise would not attend. Psychotherapy reveals how important this involvement

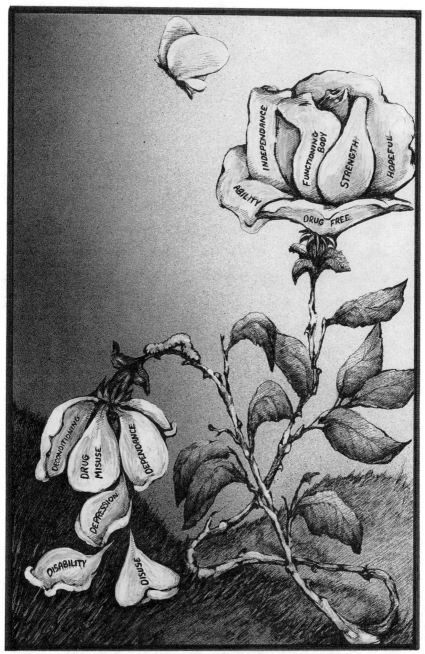

Figure 5: Patients with CBPS fight the six "*Ds*"

with her children is and leads to an agreement with them that they will continue to keep her involved in their lives even if she returns to her own home. Six months later she is back home with few complaints of pain.

Susan's pain served an important psychological function—it helped provide her with the individual attention that she very much needed. When that function was recognized and satisfied in other ways, her pain subsided.

In this chapter we've identified the key characteristics of CBPS:

1. Pain that has lasted beyond the expected healing period for that injury, illness, or condition.
2. No clearly identifiable physical condition which could cause the degree of pain being experienced, despite numerous attempts to find one.
3. No clearly identifiable medication, surgery, or physical therapy which will cure the underlying cause of the pain.
4. Significant lifestyle changes. These can be remembered by the six "Ds" described by Brena and Chapman (see references):

Deconditioning—gradual loss of muscle strength and stamina.

Disuse—not using the body or a part of the body.

Drug misuse—inappropriate use of medications leading to tolerance and drug dependence.

Dependence—on the family and healthcare system.

Lack of control over one's own life.

Depression—manifested by sleep disturbances, weight gain, lack of control. Patients often cry easily and feel hopeless. Anger is a frequent problem.

Disability—which far exceeds underlying findings and significant dependence on social and financial assistance.

Though the fate of the person with CBPS seems very discouraging, Chapters 5 and 9 will show you that there is definitely HOPE. Once the condition is clearly identified, patients can learn to live a full life again. In fact, many individuals like Joe, described at the beginning of this chapter, have been successful in changing their lifestyles to more productive ones.

Remember to take a positive attitude. Recognizing CBPS and being willing to utilize the knowledge and skills available can reverse the process of CBPS for many individuals.

KEY POINTS TO REMEMBER

Chronic Benign Pain Syndrome is persistent, nonmalignant, and is accompanied by symptoms such as depression, pre-occupation with pain, dependency on drugs or alcohol, and dependency on other people and the healthcare system.

CBPS is not just a medical issue; it also has psychological and social implications. CBPS involves significant lifestyle changes including the six Ds — *deconditioning* (loss of strength and stamina), *disuse* (of body), *drug misuse*, *dependence*, *depression*, and *disability*.

Chapter Five

KEYS: MANAGING CBPS

Karen is a forty-year-old high school teacher who has always led an active, productive life. The mother of three teenagers, she has been a loving wife and mother while also successfully pursuing a demanding career. However, her life has changed dramatically during the past year. She has come down with rheumatoid arthritis, a painful and potentially disabling condition which her mother also had. Her arthritis is controlled with a combination of appropriate drugs prescribed by her physician, an arthritis specialist who has told her the arthritis is mild and stable. However, she takes large quantities of narcotics daily and has gone from physician to physician searching for just the right combination of drugs and other treatments to relieve her pain completely. She is on a leave of absence from her job and spends many days in bed watching television. She has stopped doing the Red Cross volunteer work she loved, and she leaves most of the household responsibilities to her husband and children. Karen complains constantly and says frequently that there is no hope for her to enjoy life ever again.

A friend recommends that she try a pain rehabilitation program at a local hospital. She refuses initially because she has already seen so many doctors and received so little effective help. Finally, her husband says he can no longer take her negative attitude and constant complaining. Her school calls and says that they will have to give her position to someone else if she does not return soon. She realizes that she must do something or she will lose her family and her job. During an intensive, inpatient pain program she is able to see how her attitude is making her problem worse. She realizes that though she never may be completely free of pain, she will be able to return to her job, be a contributing member of her family, and find pleasure in life again. Karen stops taking the nonessential narcotics and other potentially addictive drugs, starts a regular walking program, and learns how to use techniques like biofeedback to help relax. Though the process of moving back into life has its ups and downs, she has learned the skills needed to cope with her pain and she actually feels significant pain relief and control over her life again.

As this example indicates, there are many problems with managing CBPS. However, with the right knowledge, commitment, and approach, chronic pain can be managed effectively. You need to understand that by manage, we mean gaining control over your pain so that you are able to be a productive person who enjoys life. We do not mean cure your pain or necessarily get rid of it forever. As this book has shown so far, chronic pain cannot be "cut out of you" as one can cut out a tumor. It cannot be tossed in the wastebasket and forgotten. It may always be with you in some degree or another. The first step in managing your pain is to accept the reality that it may always be a factor in your life.

In this chapter, we will look at various problems, medications, and therapies which you may have encountered in your search to relieve pain. Some approaches are effective with some conditions and some are not, but you will become aware of what the latest research has shown are the most effective ways to treat CBPS.

This chapter concludes with a list of guidelines which you may find useful in managing your own pain. Even though healthcare professionals can play a major role in helping you with your pain, *ultimately you are responsible for taking care of yourself.* This chapter will provide the KEYS for you to start this important process.

The process of addressing chronic pain involves many complex factors. As the previous chapter defining CBPS indicates, every facet of a person's life may be affected by chronic pain. This means that every facet needs to be taken into consideration when a chronic pain treatment program is initiated. The person with chronic pain faces many challenges.

People with chronic pain have a need to communicate with others about their suffering. Families struggle under the burden of their loved one's disability and discomfort. Just as we respond automatically to a baby's cry, we respond spontaneously to the pain of those we love. When pain persists, despite our best efforts, family members begin feeling inadequate and guilty. Sometimes they respond with irritation, denial, and withdrawal.

Healthcare professionals may be equally frustrated with their inability to alter their patients' pain significantly. Physicians want to heal, to cure, or at the least, to provide significant relief. Most physicians want to find an underlying cause and remove it. With CBPS, an underlying cause that would explain all the problems is difficult, if not impossible, to detect. Chronic pain, therefore, is frequently treated symptomatically with medications, physical therapy, and surgery.

The increase in medical specialities and the resultant fragmentation in healthcare compounds the complex problem of managing chronic pain, which requires treatment from a variety of specialists and needs a multi-disciplinary, comprehensive program. Multidisciplinary refers to different professionals with a variety of backgrounds but who share common values and philosophies in dealing with pain management. Usually one primary physician coordinates the team of specialists and directs consultation among the team members. (Chapter 6 looks at the different professionals who comprise a typical pain rehabilitation team.)

Injuries, sickness, and pain trigger responses which are not necessarily best suited for treatment of CBPS—responses such as rest, attention, and decreasing activity.

Sleep disruption becomes a particular problem to those with chronic pain. Certain drugs also interfere with normal sleep patterns.

People with CBPS feel an urgent need to search for treatment and relief. Each new treatment is approached with great expectations and frequently results in great despondency when it fails. As time goes on, hope alternates with despair, eventually leading to a change in the individual's personality and perspective on life. Bizarre proposals and drastic measures which normally would be unacceptable become immensely attractive. Thus, the stage is set for quackery.

Like Karen in the case described at the beginning of this chapter, patients with chronic pain are both desperate and depressed. Giving up sometimes seems to be the only alternative. It is only with dynamic intervention that many patients are able to gain control of their lives again.

ACUTE PAIN MANAGEMENT

In trying to plan the most effective way to treat chronic pain, we should look at some standard approaches to treating acute pain (pain which is short-term and has biological meaning) because many of these approaches are not effective with CBPS and it is important to understand why. We are all familiar with acute pain treatments which are frequently considered and sometimes attempted in the treatment of CBPS, usually with poor results.

I. MEDICATIONS

Most of the drugs prescribed for pain relief come from mainly two families—they are either aspirin-type medications or opium-type medications. Despite this fact, physicians and the public are inundated with countless drug choices with different names and in different combinations. Some are alleged to be more effective than others. This book is not meant to provide a comprehensive breakdown of available drugs, but to give you an idea of what benefits and complications may result from those you may encounter (see bibliography for more detailed references).

Aspirin

Aspirin has been used since the eighteenth century. In 1827, the active compound was isolated from an extract of willow bark and was named *Salicin*. Throughout the nineteenth century, many variations of this active compound were produced. In 1898, Bayer produced its version of the compound, acetylsalicylic acid, under the name of *Aspirin*. Basically, this same compound is still used today in many medications and cold remedies. Aspirin plays three major roles: it relieves pain, decreases inflammation, and reduces fever. Aspirin medications are categorized as anti-inflammatory drugs. Such medications which are not from the cortisone family are called "non-steroidal anti-inflammatory drugs" (NSAIDs). Aspirin is the best known drug from this group.

NSAIDs work on injured tissues or organs and have no effect on the peripheral nerves or on the central nervous system. As has been noted in Chapter 3, when a tissue is damaged, prostaglandins and other chemicals are released into the tissue causing these three indications of inflammation to develop:

1. The blood vessels are dilated; redness and warmth appears.

2. Blood vessels then leak fluid and more blood arrives, producing swelling.

3. Nerve endings are sensitized, resulting in nerve impulses which increase the unpleasant sensation called pain.

The site of the inflammation is usually red, swollen, tender, painful, and warm when touched, due to the increased circulation. Aspirin and other NSAIDs block the release of prostaglandins. As a result, the three features of inflammation do not develop as readily, and if they do occur, they are reduced.

Aspirin and other NSAIDs cause some people to have allergic reactions and develop bronchial asthma symptoms or break out in hives. The most common problem with aspirin is that it irritates the stomach and bowels and may cause bleeding. It also decreases clot formation. Very rarely, it causes severe gastric bleeding, especially in intentional or accidental overdoses. In extremely high doses, aspirin can damage the brain, liver, kidneys, and other organs.

Some NSAIDs are sometimes prescribed by physicians for pain. Trade names of a few examples are Naprosyn®, Motrin®, Dolobid®, Anaprox®, and Clinoril®. Others such as ibuprofen are available over the counter as Advil® or Nuprin®.

Acetaminophen

This group of drugs includes Tylenol®, Datril®, and Anacin-3®, which do not cause stomach irritation and are effective as mild pain relievers. How they work is not known. Excessive use or overdose can cause severe liver damage.

59

Cortisone

Cortisone/steroid hormones are the most powerful anti-inflammatory agents. They can control inflammation effectively, but they also reduce the body's defense mechanisms. Cortisone is used for selected conditions which cause acute pain, such as back injuries, and it may be used to relieve the pain from certain types of arthritis or chronic inflammation for limited periods of time. Its use, however, has to be balanced against possible negative side effects such as weight gain, decrease in immune system effectiveness, peptic ulcers, and other major complications. Because of these potential side effects, cortisone is used only for short-term symptomatic relief of most pain problems except in the care of conditions such as lupus and rheumatoid arthritis. It can be given in the form of pills, and is also effective when injected into tissues, such as trigger points or tendons for acute tendinitis.

Opiates/Narcotics

Opiates are narcotics extracted from the poppy plant that have been used since 4000 B.C. Their first use was recorded in about 1550 B.C. when a narcotic was prescribed for crying children. The Greeks called their opiate *morphine* because it produced dreams (morpheus) and also produced sleep (hypnose). Hippocrates described opium as an hypnotic (sleep medicine).

The use and abuse of opium spread throughout the ancient world from Rome. Opium was the cause of several major wars, including the nineteenth century Opium War in China. Narcotic addiction continues to plague well-developed countries, including the United States, yet opiates are also among the most effective pain relievers available. If used carefully, they can provide significant relief of acute pain; however, they are used very little in the management of CBPS because of their addictive nature and decreasing effectiveness after extended use.

As opposed to aspirin, which directly affects damaged tissues, opiates provide pain relief through their effects on the central nervous system (brain and spinal cord). In Chapter 3, we discussed endorphins and enkephalins which are naturally occurring opiates in the brain and spinal cord. These natural opiates seem to control the pathways from the brain to the painful area and have an effect on the gate control mechanism which, as explained in more detail in Chapter 3, can control the pain messages from the brain. Prescribed opiates can have the same effect.

Narcotics are commonly used in emergencies characterized by the rapid onset of severe pain. They are also used after surgery, during labor, and are very effective in terminal cancer pain management.

Many patients greatly fear becoming addicted to narcotics. Researchers point out that when narcotics are used appropriately, this fear is generally unwarranted. Though narcotic addiction certainly exists, it is usually a product of intravenous use by "mainliners" seeking the drug's euphoric effects. Patients given narcotics for injuries or terminal illness are not at much risk of becoming addicted. Narcotics do produce some unpleasant side effects, including nausea and constipation. They sometimes cause an unpleasant dream-like state. Narcotics also tend to have an effect on smooth muscles which may cause a drop in blood pressure.

The most common problem with narcotics is that they produce significant constipation. A major concern is that patients build up a tolerance which requires an increase in dose levels to generate the same effects. The amount needed to produce euphoria seems to rise much more rapidly than the amount needed to produce pain relief. A similar tendency to build up tolerance is seen in many other drugs, including alcohol.

Narcotics are effective for acute pain, but patients with CBPS should not be on long-term narcotic use. In addition to tolerance, studies of patients with CBPS reveal the development of drug dependence. If treated for a long period of time, these patients will exhibit withdrawal symptoms when narcotics are stopped, manifested by increased pain, difficulty in sleeping, shakiness, and increased sweating. Therefore, when trying to withdraw from narcotics, patients should taper off slowly or seek medical assistance with withdrawal. There is currently controversy in using narcotics for long periods of time in patients with chronic pain without cancer. Some researchers report that a few selected patients seem to increase their function with decreased pain, and without developing problems of physical dependency and addiction. However, strict criteria need to be met. My personal experience with my patients has been to the contrary. Complete withdrawal from regular narcotics is the first step in successful control over chronic pain.

Antidepressant medications

Antidepressant medications can be very effective in chronic pain management. Originally used only to treat depression, these medications have been found to produce pain relief as well. As noted in Chapter 3, the chemical theory of pain says that chemicals called neurotransmitters, such as serotonin, which is present in the brain and spinal cord, help one nerve communicate with another. When serotonin levels are low, patients become depressed and complain of aches and pains. Low serotonin levels also result in disrupted sleep.

Some antidepressants keep serotonin levels high and produce dramatic improvement in patients with chronic pain. Though antidepressants generally take from two to three weeks to have an effect on depression, CBPS patients who have been given very small doses begin to sleep more normally and their pain decreases within a few days. Though the exact reasons for this effect is not completely clear, the use of antidepressants represents a major advancement in the management of CBPS, particularly in conditions where pain seems to be produced by a nerve injury such as shingles, phantom pain, and nerve irritation from disc problems. Patients suffering from muscle pain (fibrositis, myofascial pain) also experience pain relief with very low doses of antidepressants.

Several antidepressant medications have been shown to be most effective, including the most frequently used medication, amitryptyline (Elavil®). This group of medications plays an integral role in the medical management of pain, especially chronic pain.

Anticonvulsants

Anticonvulsants are most commonly used in patients with seizure disorders such as epilepsy. Anticonvulsants seem to decrease the irritability of the nerves and consequently decrease seizures. Some painful conditions, which are considered "sensory seizures," improve with anticonvulsant treatment. It is thought that some sensory nerves continue to send pain messages to the brain and the muscles when there is nothing wrong. As explained in Chapter 3, this is one of the situations where the "doorbell continues to ring although it is not clear who is there or why." The most effective anticonvulsant drug for chronic pain management is Tegretol®, which is particularly successful in patients with severe facial pain (trigeminal neuralgia). Patients with pain from shingles also benefit from Tegrotol. Dilantin®, a medication frequently used for epilepsy, is also tried for certain types of chronic pain.

Muscle relaxants

Numerous drugs are categorized as muscle relaxants; however, controversy exists about whether muscles actually become relaxed as a result of taking these drugs. In most patients, these drugs have been very useful in treating acute pain. Valium®, a major tranquilizer, is probably the most prescribed medication for nervousness and anxiety, and it is also an excellent muscle relaxant. This has led to excessive use and abuse of Valium by patients with chronic pain. Because Valium and other relaxants produce chemical dependency and result in increased tolerance, they should not be used in chronic pain management. Other drugs such as Flexeril® and Parafon forte® are useful in many acute musculoskeletal pain problems. Used carefully, these nonaddictive medications can be used cautiously for patients with CBPS along with other nondrug approaches.

II. NERVE BLOCKS

Nerve blocks are attempts to inject a chemical into the body so that pain's pathways can be blocked. For instance, chemicals may be injected into the peripheral nerve or in the epidural space (outside the spinal cord) so that the input into the spinal cord and brain can be changed to relieve or eliminate pain. Many of these anesthetic blocks probably work through the gate theory of pain and may decrease the number of pain messages which are transmitted to the brain. Generally, nerve blocks can be divided into three types:

Blocking a peripheral nerve or a nerve root —
These types of blocks are frequently used for herniated discs, sciatica, or nerve pain, and involve injecting a chemical into the space around the spinal cord. Called epidural blocks, this approach is frequently used in acute pain management and has an immediate, albeit temporary, effect. However, a substantial number of patients report pain relief for longer periods of time—perhaps because the cycle of pain-inflammation-pain is broken.

Trigger point injections—
Trigger points are localized areas of firmness in muscle or at the bone-tendon junction. Trigger points are not only very tender to pressure, but produce pain in a different area. It is frequently a cause of persistent pain after mild muscle injuries such as whiplash or low back strains heal. If you have tendinitis or a trigger point that causes pain in a muscle, your physician may inject the sore area with a local anesthetic such as novocaine or a combination of novocaine and cortisone. The novocaine relieves the pain while the cortisone decreases the inflammation. Properly used, these blocks are very helpful in acute problems, as well as for selected patients with chronic pain.

Sympathetic block—

In addition to a nervous system which carries the sensations to the brain and motor nerves which tell our muscles to move, we all have an additional nervous system over which we have no direct control called the sympathetic nervous system. This system controls such functions as sweating and circulation. When you go out on a cold day without warm clothing, you begin to shiver. On a hot day you begin to sweat. After prolonged standing in a warm area, your hands may swell. When all this happens, you are experiencing the activities of the sympathetic nervous system. Some pain problems are felt to be caused by abnormal system activity, such as Reflex Sympathetic Dystrophy Syndrome (RSDS). This kind of pain is usually described as burning, and is associated with swelling, discoloration, coolness of the extremity, and increased sweating. Blocking of the sympathetic nervous system with a series of blocks produces pain relief in a substantial number of patients, especially in early stages.

III. SURGERY

Surgery is traditionally an attempt to cure or relieve the underlying cause of the pain. Surgery may include removal of an inflamed appendix or bothersome gallstone, or relief of pressure on nerves caused by a bulging or herniated disc. It could also involve fusion of an unstable spinal area or replacement of a damaged joint. Many new surgical procedures have been devised for management of the symptom of pain despite the fact that the underlying disease may not be correctable. These include cutting of the sensory nerves before they enter the spinal cord—a procedure called *rhizotomy*. In this approach, pain relief may occur without any loss of muscle control. Rhizotomy can be done either in open surgery or through the use of a high frequency current which burns the nerves through the tip of a needle.

Other surgical techniques include killing the nerves by using an alcohol called *phenol*. This is helpful in patients with cancer pain involving the pelvis. Two other procedures are based on the bell or specificity theory described in Chapter 3—the first in which parts of the spinal cord are cut, *cordotomy*, and a second in which a pain pathway is removed, *tractotomy*. Despite brief periods of relief, pain may recur in many patients, and new abnormal and painful sensations sometimes develop. These procedures are currently performed primarily on patients with terminal cancer pain, but not on patients with acute or chronic pain.

IV. REST

Rest is one of the most frequently prescribed treatments for pain of any kind in the acute or initial stage. In one way, it makes sense because keeping an injured body part immobilized may allow the tissues to heal; however, inactivity can lead to muscle and joint tightness and result in secondary pain and stiffness. In any case, a rest period should not last longer than a few weeks. Depending on the specific condition, movement should be encouraged earlier, especially in the case of low back pain. Only a few days of rest followed by a gradual resumption of motion is the current recommendation for acute lower back pain. Movement is essential for the health of the spine and lack of movement can create significant problems (see Chapter 3—gate theory).

V. PHYSICAL THERAPY TREATMENTS

A variety of physical therapy approaches are used effectively to treat acute pain. All of these approaches generate nerve impulses into the spinal cord and brain and can result in pain relief. It is likely that the increased circulation and warmth created by the physical modality, such as hot packs, whirlpools and ultrasound, encourage better and earlier healing. Another explanation is that the heating and cooling closes the gate in the spinal cord and prevents pain impulses from traveling to the brain. It is also possible that physical modalities may produce pain which, in turn, causes the release of naturally occurring chemicals in the brain, such as endorphins, which are known to be natural pain relievers, as described in Chapter 3.

Massage and manipulation

Massage has been used as a means of healing and relaxation in many societies throughout history. We've all experienced relief after rubbing an area that hurts. Massage, as described here, is a therapeutic technique performed by a skilled and trained physical or occupational therapist. It involves handling of tissue in a gentle way to decrease swelling and pain (stroking massage) or deep kneading of tissues, as in breaking up trigger points or scar tissue (friction massage). Massage techniques clearly help, especially to soothe tight muscles and prepare muscles for stretching. Other kinds of manipulation involving gentle twisting and pulling of tissues can provide dramatic pain relief in acute pain situations—relief that sometimes lasts for a long time. Patients with chronic pain do not, however, benefit from passive therapies in which someone else massages or manipulates the body. Self- massage may be incorporated into the patient's daily activities.

Heat therapy

In preparation for stretching and other exercises, heat is applied locally, using a heating pad, hot water bottle, or hot packs. Whirlpools can be helpful, however, they should not be used alone. Heating should be followed by stretching and other specific exercises. Patients with chronic pain may take these approaches on their own without depending on the healthcare system. A technique called deep heat (ultrasound), in which high frequency sound waves are converted to heat in the body can be used effectively to heat deeper tissues. This technique usually should be performed by trained physical therapists and should be properly supervised. Only a few sessions are necessary; prolonged, repeated use can result in dependency on these passive techniques.

Electrical stimulation

Commonly called TENS, *Transcutaneous Electrical Nerve Stimulation* has proved to be a very successful way to treat chronic pain. Working on the gate control theory, TENS involves high frequency and low intensity electrical stimulation. However, low frequency, high intensity, painful electrical stimulation works according to the chemical theory and causes the release of endorphins which produce pain relief. This is also called Acupuncture-like TENS, and has been shown to be effective in relieving pain and increasing function in patients with chronic pain. The patient can be taught to use and control the TENS unit, and if it helps to improve function and decrease the use of medications, a permanent unit can be provided.

Ice massage
Ice packs and ice massage long have been standard methods of physical therapy. Cold causes constriction of blood vessels, thus decreasing swelling, and also decreases pain in acute conditions. Working according to the chemical theory of pain, ice massage may cause endorphins to be released, resulting in pain relief. Both techniques can be learned by the patient for independent use.

CHRONIC PAIN MANAGEMENT

We've looked at the standard approaches to treating acute pain from medications to surgery and various forms of physical therapy. Some methods that are appropriate for acute pain are not appropriate for chronic pain. However, certain basic principles have been shown to work in managing CBPS. These principles have proven to be effective again and again with my own patients and with countless other patients and physicians throughout the world. After you have read Chapter 4 and determined that you have the symptoms of CBPS, you should incorporate the following important steps into your pain management program.

1. Seek multidisciplinary professional help.
Much of the advice in this book is directed toward the individual person with chronic pain and can be applied by

that person. However, very few people who have all the features of CBPS can learn to manage their pain effectively alone. The multiple problems created by chronic pain need to be evaluated by a range of professionals experienced in its management. It is sometimes very difficult for the person with chronic pain to seek this help because the healthcare system itself may make matters worse. As has been pointed out earlier, chronic pain patients typically go from doctor to doctor, searching desperately for help. Doctors prescribe medications and surgery and yet the pain persists.

Some of you who are in early stages of chronic pain or do not have all the negative effects of chronic pain may be able to apply the principles discussed here on your own. You may require help from the professionals mentioned later, while some of you may need a fully comprehensive program (see Chapter 6).

The key here is to find the right healthcare professionals, perhaps in a pain clinic setting, who are trained in chronic pain management. Chapter 6 looks in detail at these professionals and gives practical advice on how to make the right choices. You can start to incorporate many of the principles in this book into your life right away, but probably you will need the guidance and support of specialists in the field as well.

2. Eliminate narcotic and other nonessential medications.

Detoxification or elimination of potentially addictive and nonessential medications is the first step for anyone with chronic pain to take. As with Karen, whose case was described at the beginning of this chapter, you need to learn to rely on yourself to manage the pain and not to rely on these drugs. Increasingly large doses will become necessary and your whole perception of life will be clouded. Stop taking narcotic medications, such as those that contain morphine or opium, and also stop taking tranquilizers and addictive muscle relaxants.

Under professional supervision, many patients gradually withdraw from these medications by using a "pain cocktail," which combines all the medications. It is then given on a regular schedule rather than on an as-needed basis, and with gradual reduction and elimination of nonessential drugs.

Typically, when narcotics are prescribed originally, the patient is directed to take them on an as-needed basis or whenever pain is felt. However, many pain specialists feel that the individual's body responds differently after a while: instead of requesting medication when it feels pain, the body may begin to feel pain in order to receive the medication.

Gradual withdrawal is only one approach. In our program, we stop medications immediately. Side effects and withdrawal symptoms are managed appropriately through consultation with psychiatrists and *addictionologists* (physicians trained to treat addictions). Though this time of withdrawal is sometimes difficult, our experience has been that this is a successful approach for most patients.

3. Increase activity.

Through active physical and occupational therapy, the patient with chronic pain can learn to start moving again. First, trained therapists should assess the patient's limitations and capabilities, including joint range of motion, muscle strength, and muscle flexibility and endurance. Then a program of gradually increasing activity should be established. Chapter 6 looks in more detail at exactly what therapists can help a patient do. The goal is to establish an individual exercise program that can be carried out independently by the patients, so they can resume a normally active life. Patients learn the difference between *hurt*, the sensation of pain, versus *harm*, something that could damage the body. The objectives of therapy programs are to increase strength, flexibility, endurance, and general cardiovascular conditioning of the person with chronic pain. Patients learn an exercise program they should continue at home, and a flare up plan is also provided to manage any increase in pain.

4. Consider physical approaches.

With the advice of a trained therapist, the patient should consider the various physical modalities mentioned earlier in this chapter that can be used by the patient at home, such as TENS, ice massage, and heat application. Avoid passive therapies—where someone does something to you to relieve pain.

5. Increase social and recreational activities.

Moving from the cycle of withdrawal from life to participation in life is a major goal for patients with chronic pain. Rejoin your bowling league. If you can't bowl, at least you can observe and enjoy the camaraderie. If you can't jog with your neighbor as you used to, perhaps you can take a daily walk with him or her. Learning the five *P*s of pain management will help in increasing these activities (see Appendix).

6. Include family in the recovery process.

Family and friends can play a major role in returning the chronic pain patient to normal life. Consequently, families play an integral part in therapy and in educational sessions. The family needs to learn what is best for the individual patient. For a spouse, it may mean letting go of the caregiver role and giving the patient the opportunity for more independence and self-care. The family needs to be aware of what coping skills the patient is learning and reinforce them rather than reinforcing the old pain-related behaviors, such as resting, narcotic use, excessive complaining, and dependence.

7. Change negative lifestyle habits.

Certain routine behaviors may be contributing to a person's pain. Excessive coffee, alcohol, smoking, and poor nutrition can influence the discomfort of a person with chronic pain. You need to examine your lifestyle closely to determine what detrimental behaviors can be eliminated. Any habit not considered healthy for the average person, such as the behaviors mentioned here, can be devastating to a person with chronic pain.

8. Apply psychological approaches.

Various psychological approaches are used by medical professionals who work with chronic pain patients. Some of these approaches include:

Operant conditioning—This method is based on the belief that an individual's behavior can be modified by the

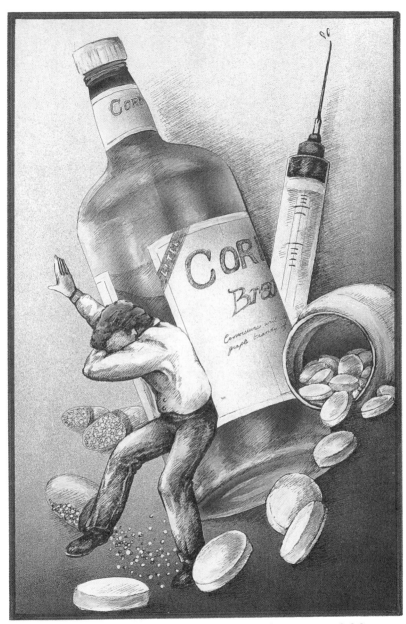

Figure 6: Medications and injections that are useful for treatment of acute pain are not appropriate for patients with chronic pain

consequences of the individual's behavior. For instance, when Karen complained about her pain and grimaced when she walked, her family paid more attention to her and she continued to be excused from her job. As a result, her pain increased rather than diminished. When her family started to leave her alone when she complained, and her employer warned her that she might lose her job if she did not return, her pain diminished. In an operant conditioning program, reinforcements are removed for pain and replaced by reinforcements for "non-pain" or "well" behavior.

Dr. Wilbert Fordyce of the University of Washington in Seattle pioneered the operant conditioning, or behavior modification approach, to dealing with chronic pain. Most pain rehabilitation programs utilize some variation of this approach successfully. This doesn't mean that the patient's pain is not real, but that by taking the focus away from pain and its rewards, a person can concentrate on more positive aspects of life.

Cognitive Restructuring—This approach is based on the belief that when patients have more information and a deeper understanding of their pain, they can change their thinking and interpret their pain differently. Patients are educated about not only what is wrong with them, but also what is right with them. Teaching the patient specific skills which help in managing pain is part of the cognitive approach. This book is an obvious attempt to educate the patient about pain and impart the skills to deal with that pain. Patients and therapists need to work together closely during this cognitive process, with a sense of trust and mutual respect.

Biofeedback—Biofeedback is a process during which patients are provided feedback about their own biological signals. Using an electronic device, patients can see how their body is reacting. For instance, they can see whether their muscles are relaxed or tense by feedback with a sound or a light. As patients learn to monitor their own body responses, they can learn to deal with their anxiety and the result is decreased pain. The gate control theory comes into play again here because the gate may be closed by the relaxation biofeedback encourages.

Relaxation training—Through biofeedback or hypnosis, the patient can learn to detect body responses and refocus his or her attention to decrease sympathetic nervous system activity and muscle contractions. Well-known researchers such as Dr. Herbert Benson recommend that patients be trained to develop their own relaxation response. Dr. Edmund Jacobson describes a progressive relaxation technique during which patients are taught to relax individual muscle groups in progression through a therapy session. Relaxation techniques appear to result in dramatic bodily changes including lower blood sugar, decreased respiration rate, and decreased anxiety. Relaxation training is particularly effective in dealing with muscle tension headaches and muscular types of pain. This kind of control over muscle tension gives confidence to some patients and seems to result in overall control of pain.

Cognitive coping skills—Patients need to learn different strategies to cope with pain. The most common is distraction. When pain occurs, we can learn to use positive imagery by conjuring up pleasant thoughts to distract us. In recent years, psychologists have devised a variety of techniques that can be incorporated into cognitive coping skills. Examples are *imaginative inattention* in which patients learn to ignore pain by imagining a situation which is just the opposite, or *imaginative transformation of pain*, in which the patient transforms the pain in his mind from a burning or a tingling to a pleasant physical sensation such as being touched gently. Other techniques might involve imagining that your pain is the result of a heroic act rather than a work injury, or focusing on an external object rather than your pain, or playing a word game in your head instead of thinking about your pain. These approaches do not work at all times with all patients, but they are skills which a patient should study in the process of learning how to manage pain.

9. Decrease depression, increase hopefulness.

Regaining a positive outlook on life is essential for the chronic pain patient. Antidepressants and forms of psychological therapy can be very helpful in this process. Techniques listed under psychological approaches may work for some people. Negative emotions which almost always accompany chronic pain need to be recognized and addressed. Fear, anger, anxiety, and hopelessness are understandable feelings but they are very harmful. Your attitude may be the most important single factor in learning to manage pain. *Pain can be either an obstacle or an opportunity.* Patients with chronic pain must recognize that their pain is providing them with a unique opportunity to confront a challenge and begin to lead a new, positive life.

With CBPS, establishing a program with the right combination of approaches for each individual is the key to success and it is difficult to do this alone. For Karen, the combination of detoxification, education, a physical rehabilitation program, biofeedback, and group therapy were the answers. Most professionals experienced in management of chronic pain will acknowledge the effectiveness of all the techniques suggested in this book. Setting up the program that will be most effective for each individual is the responsibility of professionals in the field, but it is *you*—the patient with chronic pain—who must first recognize the problem, go to the right professional, and then follow through on a treatment plan developed for you. The Pain Rehabilitation Team (Chapter 6) working with the patient determines the combination of treatments that would be appropriate for each person. *You* are the person disabled by chronic pain. And…*you* are the person who can develop the attitude and determination to become a productive, happy person again. Regaining a positive outlook on life is essential for the chronic pain patient. Chapter 7 provides more information on stress management and other psychological approaches that are useful in managing chronic pain.

KEY POINTS TO REMEMBER

Managing CBPS involves gaining control over your pain so that you can be a productive person who enjoys life. The first step in managing pain is to accept the reality that it may always be a factor in your life. There is no cure for chronic pain, but control can be achieved.

Drugs like aspirin, cortisone, and narcotics are mainly used in the treatment of acute pain and are not as effective with CBPS.

Nerve blocks, or the use of chemicals to block nerve pathways for pain, can produce relief in some types of CBPS. Surgery and physical therapy treatments, such as massage, heat, and TENS are useful for acute pain, when an identifiable problem exists.

Management of chronic pain may use approaches different from, and sometimes completely the opposite of, those used for acute pain. Progressive graded activities are used instead of rest,

KEY POINTS TO REMEMBER (continued)

tranquilizers and narcotic medications are avoided, and attention is directed toward well behaviors, rather than pain behaviors. One key difference is the use of education and psychological coping skills to apply the newly learned skills in treating patients with chronic pain.

Professionals trained in the management of CBPS will start advising you to eliminate addictive medications. Gradually, moving from a typical cycle of withdrawal to active participation in life is another major step in pain rehabilitation. Family and friends should play an important role in the process. The application of various psychological approaches such as cognitive restructuring, biofeedback and relaxation training, can also be effective.

Regaining a positive outlook on life is essential for the chronic pain patient. A person's attitude may be the single most important factor in learning to manage pain.

Chapter Six

TEAM: THE PROFESSIONALS

After two years of disabling back pain as the result of a motorcycle accident, Michael, a thirty-seven-year-old married male, decided to seek specialized help for his condition, which met the criteria for CBPS (see Chapter 4). He lived in a metropolitan area where there were several highly publicized programs which promised pain relief. Choosing the right program and professionals was extremely challenging for him. After visiting several different pain clinics, he chose an inpatient pain rehabilitation clinic at a local hospital. After consulting with his physician, it was determined that the first step in Michael's treatment would be to get him off all the nonessential drugs he had been taking to control his pain. This was difficult at first, but Michael began attending lectures and discussing the reasons for this step. He gradually started exercising, and soon he found himself stronger. He was sleeping better too, thanks to the new antidepressant medication that was prescribed. One of the best parts of the program was sharing his frustration with other patients about their experiences with pain and its effect on their lives. After three weeks, he graduated from the program and returned home. Within two more weeks, he was back at work. Whenever he started to feel pain, he used the flare up techniques such as stretching exercises, imagery, and relaxation he had learned in the pain program and the pain usually subsided. His pain was not completely gone, but he had learned how to function despite it. He felt in control of his pain and his life again.

M ichael's pain had an impact on many different facets of his life. Consequently, when he decided to seek professional help he needed many different professionals working together to help him manage his pain and the problems it had caused. Rather than going to one more doctor (after having seen more than a dozen over the last two years), he decided to enter a comprehensive inpatient program where he would be assisted by a variety of professionals.

Recently, as the devastating problem of chronic pain has become more widely recognized, more than one thousand pain clinics and pain centers have been established across the United States. These treatment centers differ greatly. Some are comprehensive facilities connected with universities or medical schools, while others are run by individual physicians in their offices. Some clinics are obviously more effective than others.

Choosing an effective program can be a challenge since no complete listing of pain clinics or comprehensive accrediting system is available. (A limited accrediting system is mentioned later in this chapter.) The original idea for a multidisciplinary pain clinic can be traced to John J. Bonica, M.D., of the University of Washington Medical School in Seattle. Dr. Bonica, an anesthesiologist, is the author of several books on the treatment of pain. He proposed that since chronic pain is a problem which affects many aspects of a person's life, it should be treated with a variety of specialists. Instead of one physician, the effective pain clinic has access to many medical and surgical specialists, as well as professionals who are not physicians, such as psychologists and physical and occupational therapists, and uses many techniques to control pain. Most patients respond best to a combination of methods such as the ones outlined in Chapter 5 on managing CBPS. These include education, physical exercises, electrical stimulation, appropriate drugs, and psychotherapy.

Unfortunately, this excellent concept has been abused by some practitioners, who have simply relabeled the same limited services they have always had without expanding their services to address all the problems encountered by chronic pain patients. The lesson for the person looking for a pain clinic is beware. Just because a program is labeled "pain clinic" does not mean it offers the multidisciplinary approach necessary to really help the chronic pain patient.

Later in this chapter we look at the challenging process of finding and choosing a pain specialist and a pain clinic; however, first we must look at the team of professionals who typically work together to handle the problem of chronic pain.

The team

As has been explained, chronic pain is a complex medical, physical, psychological, and social process. Consequently, the team which guides the management of this process should consist of professionals with specific roles. Studies have shown that when this team of individuals is functioning successfully, the impact of each professional is much greater than the effect of one specialist acting alone.

These core team members usually include a physician who is well-trained in the broad aspects of chronic pain and recognizes the unique characteristics of CBPS; a nurse; a physical therapist; an occupational therapist; and a psychologist. In addition, depending on the particular individual's needs, the team may include social workers, vocational counselors, employers, rehabilitation nurses and counselors, insurance carriers, clergy, attorneys, and others. The key is to identify all facets of the problem in the patient and then find the specific appropriate specialist to assist in that facet of the problem. One specialist, usually the physician, should coordinate the treatment process.

Physicians

The technical term for a pain management specialist is *algologist*. The physician may be trained in any one of several medical specialities. They may be an anesthesiologist, *physiatrist* (a specialist in physical medicine and rehabilitation), neurosurgeon, neurologist, psychiatrist, or primary care physician such as a family physician or internist. However, these physicians should have special training and/or experience in chronic pain management and should spend a significant percentage of his/her practice caring for people with chronic pain.

As was explained earlier, physicians without training and experience in managing patients with chronic pain often find its treatment very frustrating. Most physicians are accustomed to diagnosing a problem and then curing it, or, at the very least, relieving pain. When CBPS patients come back again and again, complaining of increasing pain and a range of other problems, the physician who is not trained in CBPS management becomes as frustrated as the patient. Chronic pain patients represent failure to many physicians—not only personally, but a failure of the healthcare system as a whole. The physician alone does not have the resources to deal with the multiple problems of a person with chronic pain. Patients with chronic pain are among the most desperate individuals a doctor will ever see.

The physician who treats patients with chronic pain needs to be compassionate and caring, and recognize that pain is a very complex and subjective sensation. The physician should never try to disprove the patient's pain. The underlying premise in treating chronic pain is that *it is real*. Medical care should focus on trying to identify an explanation for the degree of pain being experienced and then treating those conditions that are treatable. If no curative treatment is available, those areas of the patient's life that can be improved are targeted and addressed. The physician's role is to educate the patient, differentiate chronic from acute pain, communicate the concepts of chronic pain treatment, and obtain the confidence of the patient and the family in establishing a program for chronic pain management.

Physicians unfamiliar with CBPS may have much difficulty in differentiating treatment approaches for chronic pain and acute pain. A physician accustomed to seeing almost immediate pain relief after prescribing rest and narcotics will find these approaches counter-productive in treating chronic pain. As was explained earlier, acute pain therapies may actually encourage the negative chronic pain behaviors which need to be eliminated. The physician must recognize this difference.

It is very important for the physician, patient, and involved family members to build up a *trusting relationship*. The patient should feel comfortable asking for an explanation for any prescribed treatment and the physician should feel comfortable answering. Choosing the right physician is crucial in the management of CBPS. The tips at the end of this chapter provide some guidance in the important process of choosing a program and physician (see Chapter 8 for certification of physicians in pain medicine).

Nurses

Nurses play a significant role in the effective management of chronic pain. On a day-to-day basis, nurses review medication usage, provide sound nutritional advice, educate the patient about prescribed treatments, and monitor progress. In many rehabilitation programs, the nurse works closely with the physician, acting as a "case manager" and playing an advocate role for the patients and their families. The nurse may communicate the patient's needs to the team members and coordinate the team's efforts on behalf of the patient. In addition to medical nursing activities, nurses in pain programs teach rehabilitation principles and encourage self-responsibility and independence of the patient.

Physical and occupational therapists

These professionals provide the evaluation and assessment of physical problems which need improvement. They then establish an individualized exercise and general conditioning program designed to improve cardiovascular and respiratory endurance and increase flexibility, range of motion, and strength. The occupational therapist focuses on increasing the patient's ability to perform specific tasks typically necessary at home or work. These therapists have a major role in decreasing the patient's fear and building confidence through gradually increasing activity. Therapists also teach the patient how to use physical methods of pain control such as ice massage, heat therapies, and stretching exercises on their own. A flare up plan is also provided. Proper body mechanics in daily activities are encouraged.

Psychologists

Since the pain experience has so many psychological ramifications, psychologists are extremely important in chronic pain management. The psychologist first identifies those emotional conditions—such as depression, anxiety, fear, hopelessness, anger, and frustration—that have resulted from chronic pain. Then the psychologist helps the patient recognize the effects of pain and works with the patient to establish methods of dealing with the pain. The patient learns specific skills which may be very helpful, such as cognitive restructuring, relaxation techniques, biofeedback, and imagery. Psychologists provide individual and family therapy, as well as support groups that give invaluable insight and support.

Social workers

Social workers can be very effective in identifying financial, family, and social concerns which are contributing to pain-related behaviors. The social worker assesses the effects of pain on the family and may involve the family in psychological counseling or support programs which help both the patient and the family. Social workers also recommend community resources which may help the patient return to a more normal living pattern.

Many other professionals are called in frequently to assist patients with particular problems. The effective pain management program should have established a mechanism which allows for this kind of individualized approach. The most important challenge the patient and his or her family may face is to find a program which will meet the patient's complex and multi-faceted needs. The patient may be too disabled physically and psychologically to pursue this task alone. It may be up to family and supportive friends to search for the right professional help.

Others

There are many other health care professionals that may be involved, depending on your needs. In many programs, vocational rehabilitation counselors play a significant role.

These professionals have specialized training in understanding the work needs and job skills that people need to perform work activities. They work closely with the medical team, fitting the patient's physical capacities to potential job situations. Overall, the main goal in many pain rehabilitation programs is to return the injured worker, or the individual with chronic pain who is able to work, back to the same employment with the same employer. A second alternative is to keep employment with the same employer but in a different job with limitations. The third option is to consider a similar job with a different employer. Finally, the last option may require retraining in a different area and looking for a totally different job. Thus, the vocational rehabilitation counselor's involvement may be minimal in doing research for the appropriate direction, or significant, in assisting the individual to obtain the resources needed within the community for additional education, training, and finally placement in job situations.

Other members include dietitians and nutritionists. Many individuals who have chronic pain have become, as we discussed already, deconditioned. Excessive weight gain and poor nutrition are frequently seen in these individuals. The dietician's role is to counsel the patients about reasonable expectations and guide them through a successful weight-loss program. Instruction regarding proper ways of eating as well as the proper things to eat is a major task dietitians and nutritionists perform.

In many situations, other medical specialists and consultants such as anesthesiologists, neurosurgeons, physiatrists, neurologists, psychiatrists and addictionologists may be called in to help with diagnosis and appropriate treatment planning.

However it is very important to recognize that you, the person with chronic pain, as well as your family, should be an integral part of the rehabilitation team. Goals should be mutually set with a clear under-standing of the goals to be achieved, time frames, and the steps to achieve them. Only with your active involvement can significant success toward reaching these goals occur.

How to find pain clinics or pain specialists in your area

Asking for a referral from medical professionals is a good first step in locating specialized pain programs. Ask your primary care physician or any other medical professional you respect for advice on this subject. (Some pain clinics will require a letter of referral from your physician and a copy of your medical records.) You also may call your local medical or dental society (listed in the telephone directory) for the names of pain clinics and specialists in your area. Medical schools are also good sources of information. Many medical schools actually have pain clinics which are supported by the departments of anesthesiology, physical medicine and rehabilitation, neurosurgery, neurology, or psychiatry. Your local newspapers may contain announcements concerning pain support groups whose members will be helpful in recommending programs. Finally, the Commission on Accreditation of Rehabilitation Facilities (CARF) publishes a list of over 100 pain clinics which it has accredited in the United States. However, CARF only accredits comprehensive pain rehabilitation programs which apply voluntarily for accreditation. You can obtain this listing by writing CARF, 101 North Wilmot Road, Tucson, Arizona, 85711.

A neighbor, relative, or friend may also be a good resource for names of specialists and specialized programs. You will still need to evaluate a program in light of your own needs, but a recommendation from someone you trust is a good start in this evaluation process.

How to choose the pain specialist and clinic for you

Once you have identified several options, the next step is to evaluate these options based on quality and your own individual needs. When considering a physician, ask what specialized training and experience that person has had in chronic pain management. Find out what methods the physician uses to treat chronic pain. If the physician habitually uses narcotic medications and surgery as primary treatment approaches, you should look further for someone who recognizes the value of the other techniques described in this book. You also will want to stay away from a physician who does not differentiate between the treatment of acute and chronic pain.

In choosing a pain center, you may first want to make sure you are comfortable with the physician or medical specialist who directs the program, and you will want to be sure that this person has experience and training in chronic pain management. After that, look for a comprehensive program which uses a variety of professionals to treat the different physical and psychological aspects of CBPS. The clinic should also have the capability of offering a variety of treatment approaches, such as physical therapy, exercise, electrical stimulation (TENS), biofeedback, detoxification from addictive medications, use of other medications, nerve blocks, hypnosis, stress management training, and psychotherapy. Education should always be an important part of the program.

Some centers offer inpatient programs while others offer only outpatient treatment. If detoxification from addictive drugs is going to be necessary, you may want to consider inpatient treatment because you may need the intensive support usually necessary for this process. Outpatient programs are generally less expensive, less intense, and extend over a longer period of time.

A key factor in evaluating a program is determining how successfully patients transfer chronic pain management skills into their daily lives. Talk to the clinic's director about its long-term success rate.

The program that is best for you depends on your particular condition. Ask about the clinic's experience in treating your specific problem. Some programs announce up front that they specialize in one kind of condition. Headache clinics, TMJ clinics, and arthritis clinics are becoming more and more common. If the cause of your pain has not been determined, make sure the clinic you are considering offers diagnostic services in addition to treatment.

Naturally, the expense of the program is a factor, especially when financial concerns may be complicated by the patient's disability and resulting lack of productivity. It may be wise to ask your insurance company what expenses will be covered. Always make sure you understand the projected expenses before you enroll in a pain clinic program.

Programs to avoid

You will want to stay away from any program, specialist, or clinic which does the following:

Promises cures or is overly optimistic.

Regularly prescribes addictive substances on a long-term basis.

Routinely recommends surgery.

Suggests a single type of treatment for all types of pain.

Suggests that chronic pain is completely psychological or "all in your head."

Programs to consider

If the answer is "yes" to most of the following questions then you may have found the right program for your needs:

Y   N

☐ ☐ Is teaching effective pain management and not curing pain the main goal of the program?

☐ ☐ Can you enroll in the program when you want to or is there a big rush to get you in?

☐ ☐ Do the specialists you meet listen to you and respond specifically to your questions and concerns?

☐ ☐ Does the clinic have a comprehensive range of programs: evaluation, inpatient, outpatient/day program, individualized programs?

☐ ☐ Does the medical director belong to nationally recognized pain groups and participate in continuing education by attending and being involved in meetings of those organizations?

Y N

☐ ☐ Does the clinic's program involve a variety of professionals such as those listed earlier in this chapter?

☐ ☐ Does the clinic offer a variety of treatment approaches?

☐ ☐ Do you feel comfortable with the staff members you meet?

☐ ☐ Does treatment include a follow-up program?

☐ ☐ Do you sense the potential for developing a trusting relationship with the professionals you meet?

☐ ☐ Can you afford the program? Is it covered by your medical insurance?

☐ ☐ Does your physician, insurance company, or employer recommend the program?

☐ ☐ Has your physician had good results with the program?

Resources such as the International Association for the Study of Pain (IASP), the American Academy of Pain Medicine (AAPM), the American Pain Society (APS), and the Commission on Accreditation of Rehabilitation Facilities (CARF), are just some of the organizations that you can contact to obtain appropriate references for both the pain clinics and the specialists in your area (see Resources).

Summary
Traditionally, pain management has rested solely with physicians who usually have used surgery, medications, or

physical therapy approaches. Too often, the result for the patient with CBPS has been little or no relief from pain and the development of a variety of disabling psychological and physical problems. Recently, effective programs have been established which use a multidisciplinary team of professionals who work together to treat each facet of CBPS. This approach has clearly been shown to be the most effective way to manage the complex problem of the patient with chronic pain. Choosing the right professionals and the right program for the individual is the challenge; however, guidelines listed in this chapter should be very helpful in this process.

KEY POINTS TO REMEMBER

There are more than one thousand pain clinics and centers across the United States. It is important to know, however, that a program labeled "pain clinic" does not always offer the multidisciplinary approach which is essential in treating chronic pain.

The team in charge of managing CBPS at a pain clinic should at least include a physician, a nurse, a physical therapist, an occupational therapist, and a psychologist.

Your primary care physician, your local medical or dental society, medical schools, local newspapers and the Commission on Accreditation of Rehabilitation Facilities (CARF) are good sources of reference for pain clinics.

Chapter Seven

LIFE:
MANAGING STRESS

Judy was a successful thirty-five-year-old attorney with three children. Her life and career were highlighted by success after success. In addition to earning top grades, she was a champion tennis player in both high school and college. She has been on a fast track all of her life. After graduating at the top of her law school class, she was accepted in a prestigious firm where she moved up to a partnership in record time. She married an equally successful lawyer from the same firm and they had three children in quick succession. Though her days were even fuller with the demands of a growing family, she was able to balance it all and still maintain her positive outlook and pleasant disposition—that is, until the headaches started.

Judy noticed that she started having headaches at the end of the day. Sometimes they would occur in the middle of the night, waking her up and causing her to be tired the next day. Eventually, they started getting worse—sometimes lasting a whole day for no apparent reason. At first she just took aspirin and dismissed them as migraines related to her busy schedule or lack of sufficient sleep. She tried to integrate an exercise program into her daily routine, but she just couldn't keep on a schedule. Her primary care physician prescribed medications, but they didn't help. She went to a neurologist who ordered a CAT scan and an MRI (special x-rays of the brain), but there was no tumor or indication of any serious disorder.

Meanwhile, the headaches and their intensity kept increasing and her daily life was affected. She started missing days at work (unheard of up to this point). Her sleep pattern was disturbed. She became irritable with her family and her sexual relationship with her husband became nonexistent. She started going from physician to physician, searching desperately for someone who had the answer to her dilemma. One specialist told her that she did not have migraines and that she had tension headaches which would go away if she would only learn to relax. She persisted in taking codeine and Valium because they seemed to provide some temporary relief and she didn't know where else to turn.

Judy's life now in no way resembled the life she had once led. Her clients started turning to other attorneys. Her successful law practice was in a shambles and her income dwindled. She applied for disability benefits but was turned down. Medical bills were piling up. Her life was at a crossroads. She left all the cooking and childcare responsibilities to her husband who was becoming more and more upset about her condition and her inability to participate in family life. This was not the woman he married. Something was very, very wrong. Despite all the concern and all the efforts on Judy's part to solve her problem, the headaches continued.

John is forty-two years old. He joined the army right out of high school, and after a four-year stint, started working at the same foundry where his father had been employed for many years. He was a steady, reliable worker and received regular bonuses for his productivity. Within a short period of time, he was promoted to foreman. By the age of forty, he had already accumulated twenty years of seniority and was at the highest pay grade within the company. He was also active in union activities and developed good relationships with his co-workers and bosses. His health had always been outstanding; he had never needed medical attention except for a hernia repair. His one weakness was smoking—at the rate of about one and one-half packs a day—and though he knew he should give it up, he just didn't seem to be able to do it. He drank occasionally on Friday nights with his friends from a bowling league. His wife was a dietitian at a local hospital. They had three children, including two teenagers and, as far as John knew, they were "good kids."

Soon after his forty-second birthday, John was helping one of his employees lift a 150-pound basket. Because of the awkwardness of the basket, it had to be lifted onto a waist-level dock site. John twisted his back to accomplish this maneuver and felt a "pop" in his back. He almost dropped the basket, but because of his strength, was able to hold on to it. His back was sore after this incident and he went to the company nurse who suggested he go to the nearest hospital emergency room. X-rays indicated that nothing was broken and he was told that he had strained a muscle and should feel relief in a few days. However, the pain continued. Any movement seemed to aggravate the pain. He missed two weeks of work so he could rest his back and he took medication his doctor had prescribed for the pain. When the pain did not improve, he went back to the physician, who recommended physical therapy. After six weeks of physical therapy, John did sense some improvement, but after a certain point, the improvement stopped. Any increase in activity caused the pain to increase. After three months, he still was not able to return to work, and his doctor referred him to a bone specialist, an orthopedic surgeon, who repeated the x-rays. No bone problems were evident, so his doctor said John probably had arthritis. The doctor prescribed narcotic pain medications. At that point, John began to notice a pain starting down his right leg and a CAT scan revealed a bulging disc in his lower back. It was decided that his problem was not serious enough to need immediate surgery, and the doctor injected cortisone into the painful area. This lessened the pain temporarily but did not take it away completely. He started to have difficulty falling asleep, waking up many times at night with pain. He was given sleeping pills by his family doctor, but his sleep was still disrupted.

John's employer had been very supportive throughout this period. His insurance company had paid him worker's compensation benefits regularly. Although it was not the same amount as his salary, the amount was sufficient for his family to live on. However, after eight months without relief, his insurance company asked him to see another doctor for an independent medical evaluation. The new doctor suggested further tests which revealed a mildly pinched nerve. This doctor recommended that he return to light-duty work and eventually to full work.

John was very motivated since he enjoyed his work and was becoming very bored at home, but he went for one day and could not even lift a five-pound box. His back pain worsened significantly and he became very tired after one hour of working. His company sent him home.

Now, a year after the injury, John finds himself unable to sleep, waking up three or four times a night. He has gained twenty pounds and is very frustrated. He's stopped playing softball and has dropped out of his bowling league. His family did try to be supportive, but the children find their father irritable. He complains constantly. No one carries on much of a conversation with John anymore. Recently, he was persuaded by family and friends to see a psychiatrist. The doctor found him depressed and

angry. Since the physicians are finding very little wrong, his
benefits have been cut off and he is feeling financial pressures.
He has hired a lawyer who encourages him to participate in a
rehabilitation program so that he can obtain appropriate benefits.
He has filed a lawsuit against his former company and feels he
will never be able to return to his work again.

And the pain continues. John cannot stand for more than
fifteen minutes or lie down for more than an hour. Every
activity seems to make his back pain worse. In addition, he
notices that he gets headaches and becomes very fatigued after
little effort. His heart pounds when he tries to get out of bed.

S tories abound of people surmounting obstacles—of
people surviving unbelievable odds and going on to
make major contributions to their fields and to society.
Likewise, there are many people who successfully face
their pain and move on to overcome it and live full,
productive lives. Despite the seemingly desperate state
that people like Judy and John find themselves in, there is
hope for them. They can learn how to manage the pain
that is destroying their lives and find joy in living again.

The gate and chemical theories are just the tip of the
research iceberg. An explosion in pain research is
anticipated by many doctors in the field. Studies show
there is more hope all the time for people with pain, but
professionals agree that hope must come first from within.
As with Judy and John in these case studies, all the medical
breakthroughs in the world won't solve the problem of
pain if the patient is not convinced that hope is there. This

book concludes with a summary of the basic principles of pain management and with practical steps to help you in handling pain. But, first, let's look in more detail at the part the mind plays in controlling your pain.

It's all in your head!

Pain is a physical and a psychological experience. *Pain is real.* Anyone with pain knows that, or do they? Most chronic pain patients have, at one time or another, doubted the reality of their physical pain and have said to themselves, "Could all this be my imagination?" Even if they have not done that, they have wondered about those around them. Thoughts like these inevitably go through the pain patient's head:

"Does my wife really understand that my pain is real?"

"The people I'm working with probably think I'm just trying to get out of work."

"My doctor seems exasperated. He probably thinks I'm exaggerating this pain way out of proportion."

The truth is, of course, that though physical pain is real, its psychological components are real too. There are many psychological influences on pain, which can make it worse...and also make it better. Learning to integrate pain management into your life means recognizing its psychological components.

GAINING CONTROL

A sense of control over your destiny plays a significant role in your health. Psychological studies indicate that those individuals who feel they have no control over the events in their lives tend to have more illnesses. These individuals have an "external locus of control." In addition, these individuals tend to have slower rates of healing and complain of more aches and pains than the average person. In contrast, those individuals who have an "internal locus of control," or control from within, seem to be able to heal quickly and actually reverse illnesses. Even small amounts of control seem to have a positive effect.

For instance, when a child is given the choice of which arm to have a shot in, the child typically complains less about pain from the injection. Similar experiences are reflected in many other studies. Elderly people in nursing homes are happier and healthier when they are given choices about their accommodations and care. Patients with cancer who are allowed to choose their own level of narcotic medication generally consume less, show less addiction, and experience greater relief.

Sometimes, the most important factor is not how much control you have—but the *perception* of how much control you have. If you believe you can have some impact on the degree of pain you feel, then it is likely you will have an impact. Successful controllers are those who feel like the director of the play rather than the actors. Sometimes being the director means making a change. You may have to change from a physically demanding job to one that involves more paperwork. Taking control is not always easy because it sometimes means taking risks. The person who is willing to make necessary changes risks failure but also opens the door to amazing benefits. Perhaps the new job will be with different people and the work seems less stimulating. But the successful person will move forward and make the best of the new situation.

There are three keys to this success: knowledge, attitude and commitment.

Knowledge: the basis of control

Control does not evolve from belief in yourself alone but also from learning about the causes of pain and the skills it takes to relieve it. In the chapter on pain management (Chapter 5), we looked at various techniques that can work for some people—everything from biofeedback to exercise, from relaxation techniques to electrical stimulation. You need to find what works for you. What works in one situation may not work in another. Each individual needs to develop a number of effective techniques. If exercise doesn't work, then imagery may...and so on.

You've taken the first step in gaining control by reading this book. Now you have the basic knowledge to understand your pain and take appropriate steps to overcome it. This knowledge can be reinforced by continuing to read about the subject, going to support groups, and perhaps soliciting the help of a rehabilitation program designed for those with chronic pain.

Attitude: the key to continuing success

To develop a positive attitude you need to experience some success. Think about situations in your life when you thought you had no control over an event and you eventually discovered you did. Perhaps it was a hard test or class when you were in school. Perhaps you were sure you would do poorly but decided to work hard anyway—and you succeeded!

This same kind of faith in yourself can apply to your struggle with pain.

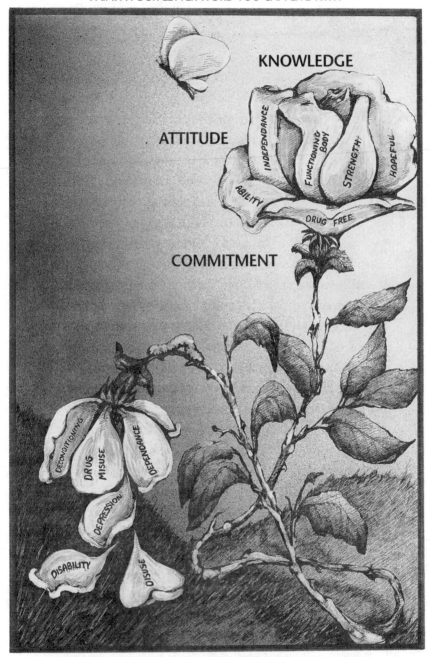

Figure 7: Features of CBPS can be overcome by
knowledge, attitude, and commitment

Frequently, particularly when struggling with chronic pain, we focus on our failures rather than our successes. We remember the last surgery or exercise program that did not work. We remember the last medication that had no effect or produced side effects. Look within yourself rather than to family members or the healthcare system for the strength to deal with your pain. Begin focussing on thoughts of the successes you have had or others who have completed their program successfully.

Commitment: essential to pain control

People who learn to live with their pain set goals and work toward them despite inevitable obstacles. They are completely committed. They don't give up. When one approach doesn't work, they try another. Commitment may be the most difficult of the three key ingredients to pain management. It is hard to stay committed when your life is falling apart all around you. It is hard to stay committed when you have tried what seems like every available resource with no relief. It is hard to stay committed when you are experiencing disabling pain. But commitment is what it takes. Once you realize that unrelenting commitment is your only hope, then the choice of whether or not to stay committed is an easy one.

Ask questions in order to establish goals

You can start to gain control by looking closely at your own relationship with pain and asking yourself these questions:

1. In what areas do I feel lack of control? Is it control over actual pain? Is it control over activity? Over medication?

2. How can I influence the areas where I feel lack of control? What kind of knowledge and support do I need to influence these areas?

3. Do I engage in the "yes, but" approach to life and pain?

My successful patients tell me that they were able to reach their goals because they got over this "yes, but" approach. Frequently, when I am trying to suggest alternatives to a patient, the response will be something like "Yes, I know that exercise helps some people, but I can't move very well" or "Yes, I know that I'm taking too much medicine, but I feel too bad when I stop." A patient takes a great positive step forward when the response is "Yes" without reservation.

4. Where am I effective and successful?

People who want to gain control first must identify those areas that they can influence. In pain clinics, successes in areas like biofeedback and relaxation therapy spill over into other areas. This is shown repeatedly in people who have tension headaches. Those with tension headaches can learn to control their headaches by relaxing muscles in distant muscle groups. When you start to gain control in some areas, you can fill up your reservoir of confidence and self-confidence and gain an internal locus of control.

5. How much control is possible? In what area? Where do I begin?

Don't start by trying to control a major event or area totally. Completely giving up coffee or stopping all smoking may be impossible immediately. But gradually cutting down according to some specific goals may be possible and will lead eventually to complete control. You could start by cutting out coffee after lunchtime and later limit your morning cups to two and then one.

These same principles apply to pain control. Expecting partial relief of pain and increasing your activities in steps can lead to more success and control. If you try to achieve all your goals at once, you are probably doomed to failure. It is important to break the long-term goal into shorter goals that are more achievable.

DEALING WITH STRESS

Stress is our emotional response to events and changes in our environment. The events themselves are not stressful— *it is our reactions to these events that generate stress.*

Stress is inevitable. Avoiding stress is not the goal since that is impossible and life would not be very interesting without some stress. Stress can be positive and can lead to creativity and positive change. However, too much stress has a physical and emotional impact on our bodies, and it definitely contributes to the intensity of pain. While lack of stress can lead to irritability, boredom, and anxiety, excess stress that is poorly controlled can lead to significant bodily changes such as migraine headaches, higher blood pressure, muscle tension, and aggravation of other pain throughout the body. Excessive stress can result in an inability to participate in normal activities.

Excessive stress, sometimes called *distress*, must be managed. The challenge, then, is not to eliminate stress but to manage it effectively.

When problems are viewed as challenges, when control is achieved from within, stress is no longer a problem but becomes an ally that will lead to increased activity and more control. Many experts compare stress to ocean waves. The experienced surfer derives a great deal of pleasure from surfing, while the inexperienced surfer may suffer great stress. Therefore, it is important to learn techniques to control and manage stress effectively so that it becomes a positive force rather than a destructive one. When allowed to become destructive, it can produce considerable psychological and physical dysfunction.

If we view the changes and events in our lives as pleasurable, then they do not produce destructive stress; however, when change is perceived as being negative, damaging stress is produced. For some people, moving to a new town may produce negative stress while others may view this change as an opportunity for growth. Then the stress that develops is energizing rather than debilitating.

The effects of negative stress have been studied extensively and there is no question about the relationship of stress and physical and mental disease. Patients with pain frequently demonstrate an excessive amount of stress. They perceive pain as totally negative, and have very little control. Holmes and Rahe have identified a scale for measuring stress. Those who are very high on the scale tend to have a much higher rate of physical illness than those who score low. Reducing stress obviously contributes to greater control over pain.

Those people who have succeeded in managing stress and in reducing pain have taken the first step of recognizing that stress is present. They understand the types and sources of stress and are committed to learning new skills for managing stress. They realize that not all stress is bad.

Types of stress

Type One stress happens when there is a life-threatening or unexpected event. A child runs into a busy street in front of your car, or you are hurrying to make an appointment or meet a business deadline. Perhaps a vicious dog starts barking and running toward you. It is likely that all these events will produce increased responses of the heart and lungs and the sympathetic system. You can actually feel your heart pounding and your breathing rate increase. You may sweat profusely and start shaking. However, this soon passes. These physical reactions in themselves are not harmful and they soon stop when the anxiety-producing event is over.

Type Two stress is characterized by a constant state of anxiety. You may be dissatisfied at work, have a tension-filled relationship with someone in your family or someone at work, or be experiencing a frustrating lack of control over pain and daily activities. You may have noticed that it's not the big things in life that really get you down. Usually we can rise to the occasion when a major crisis confronts us, but it is the little things, the ongoing frustrations, that chip away at our patience and create a continual state of stress. A person with pain lives with the constant frustration of both experiencing pain and of not being able to control pain. This person is caught up in the destructive cycle of stress. While the pain contributes to the stress, the distress increases the pain.

Stress causes chemical release

Automatic responses in the body are continually trying to combat stress. In both types of stress, the body releases certain kinds of chemicals to help us fight the stress response. In Type One stress, these chemicals can be used to help us overcome the physical reactions because there is an obvious cause and the stressful event is short-term. In Type Two stress, there is no chance for the body to recover between stressful events and it is very difficult to try to identify the specific stress.

Type Two stress builds with each small frustration. The call from your banker, a visit to the doctor, a sick child, a delay in a check you were expecting—these all contribute to a state of constant distress. There are so many small hassles that it is difficult for a person to identify which of the factors is causing the negative reactions. Each of these reactions alone is not very powerful, but in combination they can be debilitating.

When the body is aroused, it is preparing to fight or take flight. When the chemicals that accompany this state of arousal are released, bodily changes also take place that, in the case of Type Two stress where there is no immediate relief, can lead to a variety of chronic conditions such as hypertension, ulcers, headaches, and pain in various parts of the body. For the person who is already experiencing chronic pain, these physical symptoms only serve to aggravate it. Many studies in the pain field have shown that reduction of stress can decrease the perception of pain and your ability to function with pain will improve significantly, despite the fact that the exact cause of the pain is not known. Obviously, relieving stress is a necessary step.

Once you recognize that stress exists and how it works, you can concentrate on techniques to control it. You can learn these simple techniques from a professional. Most pain centers have psychologists or therapists who can give you guidelines for using these techniques. You will want to learn the following:

1. Deep breathing techniques

Shallow, rapid breathing (typical breathing in a stressful situation) decreases the oxygen supply to the brain and other vital organs; however, a simple technique of deep breathing by expanding the diaphragm (the muscle that separates the stomach from the chest) causes you to relax and relieves stress. This is a simple technique which you can easily learn and practice on your own. Put your hands on your abdomen and take a deep breath through your nose. Feel your abdomen expand to its fullest. Hold your breath for a few seconds and then breath out through pursed lips as if you are whistling. The rhythm of breathing out and in should be slow and steady.

2. Autogenic training

Although generations have known that the mind has the power to have much control over the body, this concept is still a strange one to many people, even though our grandparents always said, "It's mind over matter that counts." Scientific studies have shown that by consciously creating a pleasant vision, positive physical changes can occur. When people experiencing significant distress visualize a positive image, these thoughts affect their bodily functions by causing them to relax. Stress and pain are reduced. Autogenic training involves talking to yourself about positive behaviors. Thoughts such as "I can relax" and "I am in control" are repeated on a regular basis. The key is to focus on certain positive thoughts.

Patients who engage in positive imaging only ten minutes a day are generally more relaxed and experience less pain. Guided imagery is another way the mind can "talk" to the body. In guided imagery, you visualize a pleasant situation—such as lying on a beach listening to the waves or sitting by a warm fireplace—and a powerful sense of relaxation is induced.

In another technique called Jacobson's Relaxation Training, muscle groups are first contracted and then relaxed. The focus is on your power to have control over your muscles. Learning to have this control takes some practice and is best taught by a professional, but it can be very effective practiced on your own once you learn how to do it.

3. Biofeedback

Biofeedback is a non-invasive and painless method which helps us consciously learn to control what are normally unconscious biological functions. It is an excellent technique in stress management. There are three parts in biofeedback training:

1. Biological signals are amplified with electronic equipment.

2. The patient receives feedback and instructions from a trained professional—usually a psychologist or biofeedback technician.

3. The patient practices—initially in a small room. Later, this is all generalized in different real-life stressful situations.

With such feedback, learning of relaxation techniques can occur more quickly and efficiently.

4. Stretching

Stretching is another approach to relaxation and stress relief. When muscles are tense, a normal response is stretching. We may roll our necks, put our arms over our heads, bend forward in a chair. All these stretching movements cause us to relax.

Take a stress inventory

The best approach to relaxation and stress relief is to try a combination of these approaches. One approach will work better at one time than at another. Different approaches work better for different people. It is important to take a periodic inventory of your reactions to stress and ask yourself these questions:

What events or situations are causing stress?

How did you feel when the stress occurred?

What did you do to reduce the stress?

Which techniques were most effective for which kinds of stress?

By reviewing your accomplishments, you can learn to manage stress responses effectively. When you define the type of stress you've experienced and apply specific relaxation skills, you can learn to control stress with specific responses. Keep in mind that you don't need to avoid stress totally, but you do need to use it more efficiently if you want it to be a creative force that will energize you and help you achieve your goals.

Avoiding worry

Worry is one of the most detrimental behaviors when you are trying to maintain good health. Constant worry aggravates pain and causes us to exaggerate whatever we are worried about. Studies show that at least 40 percent of what we worry about will not happen! Realizing this and then using some of the relaxation techniques mentioned earlier to distract us from our worry are necessary steps on the path to pain relief. Revitalizing a sense of humor will help you to move beyond worry.

Humor

Humor can have a significant impact on your capacity to reduce stress. Most successful people have a quick sense of humor. They are able to look at situations from an objective perspective and find humor where others might only bemoan their fates. From the time of Freud to the present day, humor has been recognized as having a healing quality. The familiar cliche, "Laughter is the best medicine," is based on truth.

John F. Kennedy, who experienced almost continuous back pain, is a good example of a person who used humor in situations which may have been disheartening to others. (Rather than become offended when a mimic imitated his famous nasal twang, Kennedy quipped that it sounded more like his brother Bobby.)

People with chronic pain tend to lose their sense of humor—understandably, since pain is obviously not funny. I frequently hear from my patients that there is nothing to laugh about, yet it is usually possible to find humor in the most dire situations. The capacity to recapture a sense of humor is essential when attempting to live with pain. We need to recall the times when we could sit down and laugh at a joke and feel good, and then try to recreate those times.

By recognizing the psychological aspects of pain, people with chronic pain are able to use a variety of techniques to gain control over their pain and lead lives that are productive and enjoyable. Although pain may not disappear completely, it can be managed—just as people learn to manage diabetes or people with disabilities find the inner resources to go on living. Practicing stress management techniques, stopping worrying, and recapturing a sense of humor will all go a long way toward living with pain and learning to love life again.

KEY POINTS TO REMEMBER

Pain is a very *real* experience. There may be psychological components to pain but it is important to know that what you feel (or your family members feel) is real.

Gaining control over your pain is a very large part of pain management and of being a successful person in life. Knowledge, the right attitude, and commitment are the three key ingredients to gaining and maintaining control over pain.

Pain control cannot be achieved overnight, but is accomplished gradually by setting realistic goals.

Excessive stress can contribute to the intensity of pain. So, a successful program in pain management usually involves learning stress management techniques.

Stress management may involve deep breathing exercises, autogenic training (concentrating on positive behaviors), and movements such as stretching.

Chapter Eight

WHEN IS A PAIN PROGRAM SUCCESSFUL?

Adelle, fifty-three, had completed a pain rehabilitation program about six months ago. Her chronic back pain had resulted from a car accident several years before. Her pain had worsened over time to the point where she felt forced to quit her part-time job and back out on her usually active social life. This transition was very difficult for her. From an active, happy wife, mother and grandmother who walked daily, loved to dance and enjoyed her friends and family immensely, she found herself transformed into a sedentary "old lady" who winced when she managed to get out of her easy chair to turn off the television. She gained a considerable amount of weight, popped pills every hour or so, and was irritable with everyone around her. After contemplating surgery and visiting several different doctors, her family and her physician convinced her to try a pain rehabilitation program at a local hospital. After several weeks in the program, she felt much better and started getting her old self back. Her relatives started describing the program as a "success," but Adelle wasn't so sure. She felt better, but she still wasn't completely back to being her old self. After all, what is success?

Most people entering a pain rehabilitation program talk about that nebulous goal of success. But, as Adelle wondered, what is success? Just as pain is very difficult to define and not easy to explain, success is difficult to measure. There are many variables affecting the success of a pain rehabilitation program and each individual has different expectations and interpretations of pain. Unfortunately, there is no "pain-o-meter" to measure degrees of pain and to determine when pain is reduced or ceases to exist. Even if there were such a meter, a person's capacity for handling pain changes from day to day.

One measure of success for pain rehabilitation programs might be the achievement of some or all of these objectives:

1. A decrease in pain behaviors.

2. An increase in activity levels and independence in all activities of daily living.

3. Elimination or reduction of nonessential medications.

4. Improve sleep disruption and associated depression/psychological distress.

5. An increase in the patient's and family's ability to cope with pain and increase function.

6. Resumption of work or recreational activities.

7. A return to a usual social role such as worker or homemaker.

There are certainly measures other than these which are used by pain programs to assess their success, but these objectives provide a good starting point. Some of these are very subjective measures. It certainly could logically be said that if a patient's (or family's) emotional distress is lessened, then some degree of success has been achieved. The major focus is reversing the lifestyle alterations that typically accompany the experience of chronic pain and the disabilities that result.

Although one of the major goals of pain rehabilitation centers is to return individuals to gainful employment, there are several variables that are significantly related to a person's likelihood of returning to work such as the severity of the injury, and the worker's age, education, wages before injury, job seniority, availability of jobs, and economic climate.

The Commission on Accreditation of Rehabilitation Facilities (CARF), as part of its accreditation process, mandates that programs have what is called the "program evaluation system." This is a mechanism through which each program sets goals that they intend to achieve. On a three-month basis these goals are measured after the completion of the program to see whether the goals that are set are indeed achieved and maintained for at least three months. Thus, the program evaluation system measures effectiveness, as well as efficiency of pain rehabilitation programs. For further information on program evaluation, contact CARF (See Resources).

A number of studies have reported on the results of chronic pain treatment programs. One study concluded that half the patients who completed one particular pain rehabilitation program were able to return home and increase their work-related activity without taking more drugs or returning to their "pain behaviors." Other studies have supported this conclusion. Obviously, pain programs vary in their comprehensiveness and effectiveness.

Studies from major pain centers at the Mayo Clinic in Minnesota, Portland Oregon, University of Washington-Seattle, and our own results from centers in Milwaukee, Brookfield, and Sheboygan, have demonstrated the effectiveness of pain rehabilitation programs based on issues discussed in this book. From university-based settings to small community hospitals, whether inpatient or outpatient programs, positive results are being reported. Most chronic pain programs report that patients completing pain rehabilitation programs show significant drops in dependence on narcotic medications, increases in physical activities and independence, decreases in dependency on the health care system, decreases in emotional distress, increases in coping skills, and return to gainful employment. A few studies have compared treated and untreated groups and found the treated groups to show significantly more improvement. Other studies have demonstrated the cost-effectiveness of the programs. There is definitely a reduction in dependence and use of the health care system.

Programs vary in intensity (daily, three times a week), location (universities, private hospitals, clinics), type of program (inpatient, outpatient, day program), length (three to eight weeks), and cost ($4,000 to $25,000). Most rehabilitation model, multidisciplinary treatment programs are three to four weeks in length, with daily treatment (five days a week). Patients should begin to notice some positive changes in the second week. To be effective, most programs have follow-up programs and support groups associated with them. Patients' sleep patterns improve and medication dependency drops usually within seven to ten days. Activity levels increase, attitudes become more positive, and greater control over pain develops by the third week. To maintain these gains, however, patients need to continue following recommendations (see comments from patients).

So can some of these programs be termed successful and was Adelle's program a success? She had improved, but had she improved enough? Her "pain behaviors" were drastically reduced. She was more relaxed and friendlier with everyone. She stopped watching so much television and starting eating more sensibly. She still took some medications, but sometimes a day or two would go by before she felt she needed anything. She wasn't up to going out for a night on the town as she used to, but she started taking a slow-paced but regular walk around the block every evening. She even started baking her son's favorite chocolate chip cookies once in a while. But she wasn't completely recovered. She still felt pain. She

COMMENTS FROM FORMER PATIENTS

"In the PREP program, I got my caring and concerned nature and my self-respect back. I find myself feeling that at any time I can contact any of my group members or any of the staff and discuss any problem or concern I have and they will be there for me.

The staff and the group gave me a new outlook and a new chance at my life. My outlook on life was always there, but my pain just wasn't allowing me to see it.And now all I can see is a long, happy, and fulfilling life because pain is no longer a significant part of it.

All I can suggest to the new and future PREP patients is to give the program a try, a two hundred percent try, because the rewards will speak for themselves."

—Gary S. Mielke

"It has been years since I have felt this good. I can once again laugh at and with my daughters and my grandson. Life is good again.

In four weeks, I feel 200 percent better. I danced at a wedding and haven't done that in years. I wrestle on the floor with my grandson now. My 15-year-old daughter can't believe I have a sense of humor. She's telling people she never heard me laugh like I do now."

—Diana Mrozinski

COMMENTS FROM FORMER PATIENTS

"By the third week I was beginning to feel progress. I was able to do things that I couldn't do before. I was taking a lot less medication. By the fourth week I was telling myself I wanted to get back to work again. One week after I completed the pain and rehab program, I went back to work....It took a lot of determination and hard work to achieve my goal, but now I am reaping the rewards."

—Roger Hammes

"I saw people who had not worked for months or years making plans to return to their jobs. I saw people who could not return to their old jobs planning excitedly for new careers. I saw the unrestrained joy of a father able for the first time to play catch football with his son."

—Vince Calder

"The secret to success has to come from within. The ownership on making something positive happen falls on the individual.

Keep your progress in perspective. Take pride in small advances. Be satisfied with small steps. The true measure of one's progress should be measured on a monthly or yearly basis, not daily or weekly."

—Ray Ellis

couldn't imagine going back to work. Was her rehabilitation program a success?

Most professionals in the field of pain rehabilitation would say "yes!" Very few people are ever actually cured of chronic pain so the complete absence of pain is not a realistic goal; however, the reduction of pain and the ability to resume normal, productive, pleasurable activities is a realistic goal. That's why this book is called *Pain: A Four-Letter Word You Can Live With*. Adelle was learning to live with her pain and that can certainly be described as success. But Adelle, herself, will have to decide if her rehabilitation process actually meets her own personal criteria for success.

Other patients will have to go through the same process and, because people have different thresholds of pain and different expectations, their interpretations about what is successful will also be different.

If significant improvement can be defined as successful, then Adelle's program was definitely successful. In any case, her efforts in the pain program were certainly worthwhile because she has taken many positive steps toward leading a more enjoyable, normal life—she is literally learning that "pain is a word she can live with."

I also emphasize that while it is important to learn to live with pain, improved function despite pain is the goal of a pain rehabilitation program. Most of our patients have indeed increased function through returning to work and dropping their dependence on family and the health care system. Thus, effective pain management programs prevent and reverse disability.

At the beginning of each chapter, this book introduced a composite patient. All of these are based on real success stories—patients who have accomplished what they, their families, and their physicians had thought was impossible. They set goals and achieved them. I hope you have similar success in applying the knowledge in this book and find a health care facility and physician to assist you and your family in achieving the realistic goal of improving function—despite pain.

Chapter Nine

HOPE: LEARNING TO LIVE WITH PAIN

This book has presented the approaches you need to learn in order to live full, productive lives despite your pain. This final chapter will summarize and highlight what you have learned so far. The points outlined here summarize the principles of a sound pain rehabilitation program. If you keep these concepts in mind and organize your pain relief program around them, you will have taken a major step on the road to successful living again.

- Chronic pain is different than acute pain. It needs to be treated differently. The standard approaches to acute pain treatment, including rest, medications, and surgery, do not usually work for chronic pain.

• Chronic pain seems to be more common in wealthy societies—perhaps because these societies provide reinforcement or incentives for the continuation of pain. Eliminating these incentives may make pain relief and productive living more likely.

• Opiates or narcotics, which are used frequently and regularly in the treatment of pain, can be very destructive for patients with chronic pain. Antidepressants have been a great boon to pain management, especially in selected chronic pain patients.

• The mind plays an important role in the control of pain. An increased understanding of how pain works is essential if you are going to learn to control pain and lead a productive life. You need to develop a respect for the capacity of the mind to gain control over pain and have a major impact on pain relief.

• Chronic pain is frequently too complex a problem to tackle without professional support. Working with an experienced health professional or with an effective pain rehabilitation program is invaluable for many people.

These principles lead us to specific steps which can be taken in learning to live with pain and find pleasure in life again. When you first try to manage your pain, you may need to read through these steps several times every day so that they are integrated into your daily life. (Note that there is a tear-out page at the end of this book with these steps on it. Keep these principles with you and refer to them whenever necessary until you start to have control over your pain.)[1]

1. Accept the fact that you have chronic pain.
Many people become preoccupied with finding a cure that does not exist. If you accept the fact that pain will always be part of your life, then you can integrate pain management into your daily activities and go on with living. Patients with diabetes, emphysema, and other conditions that cannot be cured, have learned to control them and improve their functioning, and patients with chronic pain can learn to do the same.

2. Set specific goals in your work, recreational, and social activities.
When you set goals unrelated to your pain, your focus moves from pain to productive activities, leading to a more positive attitude and the ability to achieve these realistic goals.

3. Direct your anger at the pain.
Instead of becoming angry and irritable at the people around you, use the pain as the target of your anger. This

1 *Mastering Pain: A Twelve-Step Program for Coping with Chronic Pain* by Dr. Richard A. Sternbach, Director of Pain Treatment Center, Scripps Clinic and Research Foundation, Lajolla, CA.

way, pain won't control you and you will have more of an incentive to overcome it and move on with your life.

4. Stop taking all narcotic drugs.

You may need to decrease your drug dosages gradually; eventually, however, regular use of addictive medications must be stopped completely. Your tolerance for drugs increases as their use continues, making them virtually ineffective.

5. Focus on achieving good physical health.

Avoid stimulants such as caffeine and nicotine. A regular exercise program is vital to both the mind and the body. Stretching and moving seem to keep the "gate" nourished with positive influences, diminishing the amount of pain which goes through the gate.

6. Learn relaxation techniques and then practice them.

Practice relaxation techniques every day. Learn to identify your body's signals for stress and then apply these techniques.

7. Balance your activities. Learn to pace yourself.

Take regular relaxation breaks and switch from one activity to another. Also avoid too many activities at one time (Figure 6).

8. Seek support—not sympathy, from your family, friends and co-workers.

Make it clear to everyone that you prefer praise for your accomplishments rather than a focus on your pain and disabilities.

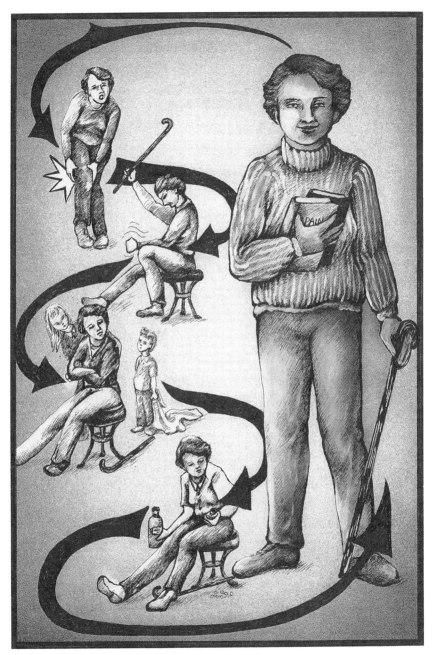

**Figure 8: Regaining control over your pain
and your life**

9. Don't expect your doctor and the healthcare system to provide all the relief you seek.

Pressuring your doctor for a cure only causes anger and frustration on your part—and the doctor's part.

10. Seek out experienced, supportive, professional help.

Find a doctor or other health professional who understands the complexities of chronic pain and is willing to support you in your efforts to handle your pain. You may want to consider a pain rehabilitation program such as those described in Chapter 6.

The choice is yours. What do you choose—to live with pain that completely disrupts your capacity to enjoy life or to move forward despite your pain, and live a productive life again? Using the techniques and approaches outlined in this book, you should be able to gain control of your life and experience a significant decrease in your pain. No one can promise you total pain relief; however, you will be able to love, laugh, enjoy your family and your work, if you have faith in yourself and are committed to your own happiness.

I hope this book has given you a sense of optimism. The title was selected because pain is indeed a four-letter word. The connotation that four-letter words are negative and bad is very common in the general public. This book, however, contains many four-letter words such as care, love, live, hope, and team, which are essential parts of the overall approach to pain management.

It will give you a better understanding of your problem. Continue to seek the best medical research. Trust your physician and work closely with your healthcare team. I wish both you and your family the very best of luck in your endeavors in pain management.

EPILOGUE

"I am Special"

The following acronym outlines many of the keys points of this book:

I is for information regarding pain, the gate and bell theories, drugs, and other issues related to chronic pain.

A is for alternatives for treatment: i.e., the medical surgical, physical/psychological/psychiatric.

M is for medications—the importance of taking the proper medication in correct amounts, for the ideal purpose and for the right period of time.

S is for surgical treatment. If and when appropriate surgical interventions are needed should be discussed with your surgeon.

P is for physical exercise and pacing activities.

E is for emotion and how it relates to pain. Increased anger, anxiety, and frustration all increase pain. By using autogenics and relaxation therapy, emotion can be reduced and pain therefore minimized.

C is for clinics/counselling.

I is for insight and incorporating knowledge in day-to-day activities.

A is for activities—the importance of staying active and avoiding deconditioning.

L is for living a productive and functional life without dependencies upon others.

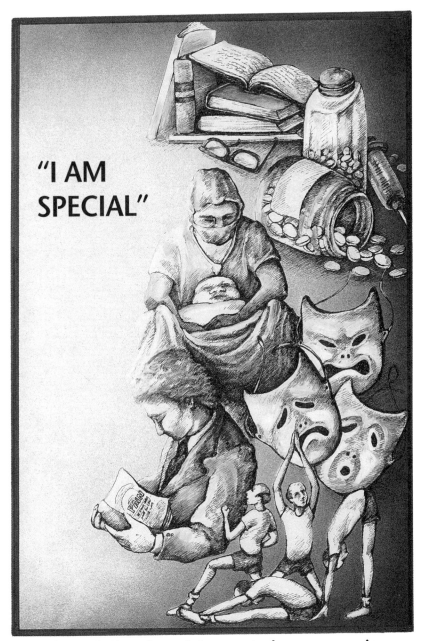

Figure 9: Keys for gaining control over your pain and your life

Appendix

PREP/CPWR— COMPREHENSIVE PROGRAMS

The appendix discusses two programs I have been associated with that are designed to help individuals with chronic pain. You currently may be participating in a program, or considering one. The information in this book should help you get the most out of the program through giving you an understanding of the rationale of the techniques used. Not all programs offer the same or similar treatments, but rehabilitation programs dealing with patients with chronic pain may incorporate some or all of the processes described herein.

Background

Just over thirty years ago John J. Bonica, M.D., a professor of anesthesiology at the University of Washington in Seattle, established the first recognized, comprehensive, multidisciplinary pain clinic. Much has transpired in this field since then and the number of such clinics has increased significantly to meet the needs of those with chronic pain. The underlying rationale for the treatment of chronic pain in a pain clinic is the recognition that it is a multidimensional problem. Coping with this problem requires a physician with a broad understanding of the facets of pain and the resources of additional physician specialists and allied health professionals, including psychologists, physical and occupational therapists, nurses, social workers, and others to comprise a team. This team works synergistically so that the sum of team members working together produces a better result than these individuals working alone—much like a symphony orchestra made up of numerous players with different instruments who produce a result together that no individual can accomplish alone.

The words pain clinic denote different things to different people. To some it is a building, or part of a building, where a group of professionals meet and where certain services are offered. Typically, an anesthesiology department in a hospital or university may house the pain clinic. To others, it means a very specific treatment program that is provided in a structured package despite the needs of the individual. Unfortunately, some pain clinics provide only specific treatments such as physical therapy, nerve blocks, or biofeedback. In clinics such as these, the benefits of a multidisciplinary team are not obtained.

Pain clinics can be solely inpatient or outpatient, or both. Sometimes they are associated with hospitals; others are conducted out of physicians' offices or in multi-physician clinics. Some pain clinics associated with universities and medical teaching institutions provide a comprehensive range of services, and in addition to conducting ongoing research they are involved in teaching professionals how to manage chronic pain. Thus, it is difficult for consumers to identify which pain clinic best suits their needs.

The Ideal Pain Center

Such a center should encompass the following:

1. *Both evaluation and treatment services, readily available to those in chronic pain.*

2. *Inpatient, outpatient, and individualized programming.*

3. *Easy accessibility for patients and their families.*

4. *Clearly-stated criteria for admission and discharge.*

5. *A medical director knowledgeable and experienced in pain management.* The physician may have trained in any specialty but he or she should have broad-based experience in working with the rehabilitation team, and should be a member of either a regional or national pain society, as demonstrated by attendance and presentation of papers at national meetings. The physician should have a minimum of three years experience in caring for those with chronic pain.

6. *Associated physicians with different specialties who can be consulted as the need arises.* Available doctors should include, but not be limited to, specialists in

anesthesiology, neurology, orthopedics, psychiatry, neurosurgery, and internal medicine and its subspecialties.

7. *Other readily available services.* These should, as needed, include pharmacy services, psychological evaluation and treatment, rehabilitation nursing, physical and occupational therapy, social services, and vocational rehabilitation. In addition, recreation therapy, spiritual counseling through chaplaincy, and other support systems should be available.

8. *Ongoing research activities and community education about pain.*

9. *Accreditation by organizations such as the Joint Commission on Accreditation of Healthcare Organizations (JCAHO) and CARF (Commission on Accreditation of Rehabilitation Facilities), voluntary accrediting bodies.* The latter has developed standards for chronic pain rehabilitation programs through national consensus of their advisory committees. CARF can accredit both inpatient and outpatient programs.

10. *A program manager in addition to the medical director.* The holder of this position should be available to discuss the pain program with the patients, representatives of the community, and referring sources. The program manager should serve as an advocate for the patient.

11. *An affiliation with a university or teaching hospital.* This indicates that the professional staff is active in teaching and research as well as in providing clinical services. This may not be available with all programs.

(Please refer back to Chapter 6 where questions are provided to help you set guidelines for selection.)

Successful management of chronic pain requires a partnership between the physician, the team of professionals, and the patient. It is important to match the physician's qualifications and style with your own. There are times when you must be assertive and discuss your needs with the professionals so that they can meet your concerns.

The Pain Rehabilitation and Evaluation Program (PREP)

This program is located at Elmbrook Memorial Hospital in Brookfield, Wisconsin, and began accepting patients on January 5, 1985. The program was designed to provide comprehensive evaluation and rehabilitation for those individuals whose lives are disrupted with chronic pain. It started out small with a maximum capacity of four patients, predominantly enrolled on an inpatient basis. It now has the capacity to care for eight to twelve patients on both an inpatient and outpatient basis.

In 1989, the program's name was changed to the Pain Rehabilitation Center. The center provides treatment to both inpatients and outpatients, utilizing a structured, comprehensive full-day program and individualized treatment programs. In addition, the Pain Rehabilitation Center has the ability to provide both screening and an outpatient evaluation for patients with chronic pain and their families.

As medical director, I have been associated with the program at Elmbrook Hospital since its inception and I continue to be active in this role. In this chapter I will explain this particular program and how it works. (Readers, however, are asked to contact the most appropriate facility in their communities, and by using the checklist at the end of this chapter as a means of assessment, to determine whether or not a specific program can provide the type of services and resources that are needed.)

Although over 75 percent of our patients are referred to the Pain Rehabilitation Center at Elmbrook Memorial Hospital by their physicians, insurance carriers are increasingly initiating referrals through their rehabilitation nurses. Approximately 5 percent of referrals are self-initiated by the patient or the family.

The initial contact is by telephone with the secretary or the manager of the Pain Rehabilitation Center. The representative of the program tells the prospective patient about the pain rehabilitation program's policies, procedures, and criteria and takes information concerning the patient's diagnosis and areas of concern.

The next step in the process is a *pain screening evaluation*. Over 80 percent of our patients undergo the screening process, which consists of an evaluation by me, a physiatrist (a physician specializing in physical medicine and rehabilitation), and a psychologist. During the screening the patient is also interviewed by the manager or designate of the program or the nurse-case supervisor, one of whom describes the elements of the program to the patient. A pain questionnaire, designed to obtain as much information as possible about the patient's problems before he or she is seen by the professionals at the pain center, is filled out. Whenever possible, all previous medical records are obtained prior to the first visit.

The examination by the physician consists of obtaining and reviewing the details of how the pain started and what has been done for it thus far. A complete review of any medical records is conducted, and the patient is examined thoroughly. The area or extremity involving the pain comes under scrutiny. Over an hour is set aside for the first interview to allow time for discussion after the history is taken and the examination done.

Milwaukee Approach

I utilize a technique I call the "Milwaukee Approach" in my discussions with patients. I have found this to be very helpful in my practice. Essentially this process involves the following:

M = *Milieu, or the environment.* It is important to establish a positive, caring, and comfortable environment where discussion can occur. After the examination I sit down with the patient and the members of his or her family or support system to discuss my findings. I tell the patient about my background and why the patient was referred to see me.

I = *Information.* I try to obtain as much information from the patient as possible. I attempt to find out what the patient knows about the pain problem, and the two most frequent questions I ask are, "What do you think is causing your pain?" and "What do you think should be done about it?" The typical answer I hear is, "I don't know. You're the doctor—you tell me." I persist in trying to find out from the patients what they think, probing for any information that may have been given in the past. In this way, I can clarify any misconceptions patients may have and give them correct information obtained from the physical examination and their medical records.

L = Label. Patients frequently are given multiple labels or diagnoses which confuse them, or they are given no diagnosis at all. I attempt to clarify the medical diagnosis and explain its meaning. I discuss the role of psychological factors that affect pain, especially if a significant element of depression appears to exist.

W = Why? In this section I try to answer the patient's questions about why he or she has continued problems with pain despite the passage of time and seemingly adequate approaches to treatment. We discuss the differences between acute and chronic pain and the psychological, social, and environmental factors that may be aggravating the patient's perception of pain and the lack of control over it. The rationale for the diagnosis and the treatment done so far are discussed here, as are suggestions for the future.

A = Aims. We discuss the broad aims we hope to achieve, and the long-term and short-term goals along the way. For example, patients are informed that the goal of managing chronic pain is not to *cure*, but to *cope*. The skills and information necessary to accomplish this goal are discussed.

U = Understanding. I explore the patient's understanding of the concepts we have presented, and take this opportunity to deal with any confusion that may have arisen concerning the information discussed so far.

K = Knowledge. We discuss additional ways of understanding pain. A brief exposition of the doorbell theory and the gate theory is presented to the patient. I present further details about the program and the principles of pain management. The use of antidepressant medications and the rationale for discontinuing addictive medications are discussed.

E = *Engage in Feeling.* I ask the patient what his or her response is to the information we've provided so far. Some are pleased to discover that there is hope. Others are angry due to their perception that the pain program does not understand their pain and does not recognize that the pain is *real.* I try to deal with their anger and frustration by clarifying the information.

E = *End.* We terminate the interview after a reasonable time. If some questions are left unanswered, I ask the patient to write them down and bring them to sessions of the program for discussion.

Next, a psychologist evaluates the patient by means of an interview and a variety of pencil and paper tests. This assessment determines what psychological factors may be affecting the patient's ability to control pain and evaluates psychological changes that have occurred during the time the patient has had chronic pain.

The nurse or the manager explains the components of the program and the need for the patient's active participation. Insurance information and additional medical records that are needed are obtained.

Team Conference

The screening team, including the physician, psychologist, and manager of the program, meets in conference. The patient, members of the patient's family, and representatives of the insurance company are invited to attend. At this conference the decision is made as to whether or not the patient will be admitted to the program. One of the following conclusions may be reached:

- To admit the patient to the inpatient program.

- To admit the patient to the comprehensive, full-day outpatient program.

- To provide individualized pain rehabilitation.

- To send the patient back for additional evaluation and/or appropriate medical or surgical treatment.

- To discharge the patient, as he or she does not meet the criteria for the program. If referral to another program is needed, this is done.

Following acceptance into the program, a review of the patient's insurance coverage is conducted by the manager. Patients are informed clearly about the cost of the program and their financial responsibility.

After a patient enters the program or if a full outpatient team evaluation has been requested, the evaluation will include:

A. A *physical therapy* assessment, to ascertain what limitations exist to strength, endurance, range of motion, and function and to develop an appropriate plan to improve deficiencies.

B. A standardized activity test termed the *EPCAT* (Elmbrook Physical Capacities and Activities Test), that measures the minimal level of functional activity. A maximum number of 84 points can be obtained on this test and patients are measured against this number. Most of our patients make average scores of only 25 to 40 on their initial assessment. By the time they complete the program, almost everyone scores 84.

C. An *occupational therapy* evaluation that assesses range of motion, strength, and the ability to carry on activities associated with daily living (ADLs). These include self-care activities, such as dressing and personal hygiene and homemaking activities, such as cleaning and cooking. Any limitations due to pain are noted, along with recommendations for improvement.

D. A *nursing assessment* to review the patient's medical status and details a nursing diagnosis and care plan. Medications taken for pain are noted, as are other medical and psychosocial factors that affect patients' ability to care for themselves.

E. *Other appropriate specialty assessments*, which could include consulting an addictionologist, if dependence on medication is suspected. An assessment by a psychiatrist, if significant psychological factors seem to be affecting the patient's ability either to cope with pain or participate in the program, may take place.

Following completion of this comprehensive assessment, a team conference is conducted and a recommendation made as to the individual's suitability to participate in the program.

The Program

Patients who have been evaluated by the screening team or the full team and found eligible for the inpatient or outpatient aspect of the program are then admitted. Admission typically takes place on Monday morning or Sunday night for inpatients.

The patients who previously had only a screening evaluation will undergo the rest of the team evaluation in the first twenty-four to forty-eight hours. Each Wednesday morning, a team conference is held to assess progress and newly admitted patients who have completed the full team evaluation are discussed again to see if it is appropriate for them to continue with the program.

Figure 10 shows the typical schedule the patients in our program follow. Most of the program is carried out on a group basis; however, the patient's program is also personalized. If it appears that a patient needs individual instruction in biofeedback or physical therapy, or private counseling, these activities take place at the end of the day.

The patient is formally admitted to the inpatient program by a primary care physician. Sometimes the patient's own doctor may be on the hospital's staff and will admit the patient. In other cases, a primary care physician on the Elmbrook staff assists us by performing complete physical examinations. During the hospital stay, this physician manages any medical problems the patient may have or may develop. Many of our patients have high blood pressure, heart disease, or diabetes, and their medical status and medications must be monitored closely.

Patients are seen regularly by me to monitor the goals and achievements of the pain rehabilitation program. All the techniques discussed previously come into play and are applied as needed.

Our program is educationally oriented. More than thirty-five hours of didactic lectures are delivered to patients and their families. I personally lecture on the different theories of pain, how to differentiate between

	Monday	Tuesday	Wednesday	Thursday	Friday
7:30	Nursing assessment and daily monitoring				
7:45	Breakfast		Breakfast	Breakfast	
8:00			Staffing		
8:30	Morning exercises			Morning exercises	
			Morning exercises		
	With physical and occupational therapy				
10:30	Open				Nursing education
11:00	Group psychology				
12:30	Lunch		Graduation	Lunch	
1:00	Individual appointments	Nursing education	Lunch	Occupational therapy education	Therapeutic recreation
1:30		PT education	Dr. Vasudevan's lecture		Aerobics
2:00	Aerobics			Aerobics	Group OT
2:30	Group occupational therapy		Family group psychology	Group OT	
3:00	Relaxation group	Individual biofeedback		Individual appointments	Open
4:00	Open		Open		
4:30	Therapeutic recreation outing	Open	Therapeutic recreation outing	Open	
5:00					
5:30		Dinner		Dinner	Dinner
6:00		Exercise quotas	Exercise quotas	Exercise quotas	Exercise quotas

Figure 10: A typical schedule for a patient in a pain rehabilitation program (Elmbrook)

acute and chronic pain, managing low back pain, and understanding and treating myofascial pain. In addition, each team member holds significant educational and informational sessions. The physical and occupational therapists review what the patients have learned about the lower back: how it works and what techniques to employ to avoid a recurring pain problem in this area.

Patients are instructed in physical techniques to control pain—*nonpharmacological methods*, as they are commonly termed. The uses of ice, cold packs, hot packs, and stretching exercises are taught. The psychologist teaches relaxation techniques, and in some situations, provides individual biofeedback instruction. We encourage the patients to employ these techniques rather than medications for pain when a symptom first becomes apparent.

The patient is also taught the difference between *hurt*—a symptom of pain, and *harm*—something that may cause damage. The patients are given certain restrictions based on their underlying medical problems, if any, and are asked to work within these restrictions toward a certain level of activity in preparation for a return to work. We may try physical techniques, such as transcutaneous electrical neurostimulation (TENS). The exercises, which include brisk aerobics, help by increasing flexibility and cardiovascular endurance. We teach the patients the doorbell theory and tell them that even though the bell is ringing, there is no one at the door. We provide them with mechanisms which will enable them to ignore it.

We also teach the patient a *flare-up* plan, usually in the last week of the program. We have found that patients might experience flare-ups after they finish the program—recall that we are focused on coping with pain, not curing it, and therefore pain symptoms may recur. We give patients skills and knowledge that they can apply. In the event of a flare-up, we advise using the Five P's—Prioritizing, Planning, Pacing, Positioning, and Problem-solving.

1. *Prioritizing*—It is important for the patient to set priorities for activities which may produce the pain. A patient with bad knee pain, who has pain every time he plays tennis, may need to put it into perspective, and decide not to play the game that seems always to aggravate his hurt/symptom. Another individual with chronic low back pain who has undergone surgery for disc problems may have to find a suitable recreational replacement for the bowling she loves. These decisions become more difficult when working for a living or maintaining a household makes physical demands. In these cases, go on to the next step.

2. *Planning*—This step involves reviewing carefully the steps needed to perform the activity. Instead of jumping into it, spend some time preparing for it. Acquiring better equipment, such as a good vacuum cleaner to make caring for a house easier, is an important part of planning.

3. *Pacing*—Patients have to accept that they may be able to carry on an activity for only a certain period of time before they must rest. After vacuuming one or two rooms, for example, the patient may decide to take a rest break before continuing instead of doing all six rooms at once and experiencing symptoms of fatigue and pain as a result. Pacing is one of the hardest things for most patients to incorporate into their day-to-day lifestyles.

4. *Positioning*—It is important to use proper body mechanics. Many patients move awkwardly and it is interesting that most of us are able to get along without much pain despite the fact that we have always used improper body mechanics. For example, carrying objects close to the body puts less stress on the back than holding the object farther away. Picking up a child from a playpen or a bag of groceries from the floor should be done with the knees slightly bent, rather than straight. Using the wrist and fingers in repetitive activities causes less strain if the shoulder and elbow are supported. Placing the body and joints in the best position gives muscles the best lever system to use the body most efficiently.

5. *Problem-solving*—This is the most important step in the event of flare-ups. If a symptom recurs, the patient needs to ask himself what it means and what the options are. The patient could go to the physician. What would the physician do? Would more x-rays show what is causing the pain when innumerable others haven't? Is more medication really the answer? Many of my patients have have had to discontinue taking medications which produce dependence. They do not want to resume narcotics, but the prudent use of aspirin-type medications may be very helpful. Should they see a surgeon? Obviously, if a symptom changes, especially if it becomes much worse or very different, or a new symptom develops, then consulting a surgeon once again will be beneficial. Many times, however, symptoms can be aggravated without a major change in the underlying problem. Nothing new can be ascertained by a physical examination or x-ray, so my patients are apt to turn to nonpharmacological approaches, such as heat, stretching, gentle exercise, and relaxation therapy.

In the event of a flare-up, physical activities are cut in half (patients are told to do only fifty percent of what they have been doing), but they are told to avoid complete rest. As soon as possible after the pain subsides or comes under control, the patient resumes physical activity and builds it up to the previous level.

Team conferences

During the time each patient is enrolled in the program, a weekly conference takes place to discuss his or her progress and status. All the team members: the physician, nurse, psychologist, and the physical and occupational therapists, take part. Pertinent information from the recreational therapist, who works with the patient twice a week, is noted, as is information from members of the patient's family. Patients (and their family members) are invited to attend the conference. Weekly progress is reviewed, and the patient's ability to achieve stated goals and move toward accomplishing his or her total goals is discussed.

We expect patients to be able to understand and accept many of the new principles we teach them, and we expect them to incorporate these principles into their day-to-day activities. If this carry-over is not demonstrated and if the patient is unable to accept any of the program, he or she may be discharged from the program.

Additional goals may be established at team conferences. As they begin to gain control over their pain, patients often show a desire to make other positive changes in their lives. Many succeed in losing weight, stopping smoking, and other personal goals.

The team conferences allow us to monitor the patient's progress and individualize the treatment program for each one. Although an average program lasts three weeks, it is tailored to each individual. Many find they require only one or two weeks of the inpatient program before they switch to the outpatient program. Others may need four weeks of inpatient programming. There are those who are able to control their pain successfully after two weeks in the outpatient program.

Goals of the program

The major goals are:

1. *To eliminate all nonessential medications.* Typically we find that 30 to 50 percent of our patients are abusing narcotics. Darvocet®, Tylenol–3®, and Percocet® are the most common. Some of our patients use tranquilizers too—typically Valium® and Xanax®. Although in the past we have used the "pain cocktail" method, in which medications are given on a timed basis rather than on demand, for the past two years we have successfully used the services of an addictionologist. These physicians, who specialize in helping those addicted to a variety of medications, have developed new techniques to help people stop taking all narcotic and addictive medicines. This is usually accomplished during the first week, and the long-term results have been encouraging. Patients dependent on and misusing medications (including alcohol) frequently need an inpatient program.

2. *To improve sleep patterns and control depression.* Sleep disturbances affect 85 percent of the patients referred to our program. When this problem is severe it is usually accompanied by mild to moderate depression. These

patients are often admitted to the inpatient program, because it has the ability to give medication on an individualized dosage and to address any side-effects which may occur. A quarter of the normal dose of an antidepressant medication such as Elavil®, Sinequan®, or Desyrl® often provides significant help with sleep problems and other depressive symptoms. If the depression is deep, we consult a psychiatrist who assists with the medication adjustment. Typically, patients find they have regained control of their dysfunctional sleeping in ten days to two weeks. Depressive symptoms also seem to improve greatly by the end of the second week. At the end of the program, these patients are being maintained on a low dose of an antidepressant medication. Most wean themselves from it gradually in the next four to twelve weeks.

3. *To increase physical activity, flexibility, and endurance.* Patients receive a quota of exercises in a graded physical occupational therapy program. They start at a level under which they can perform comfortably, then this is built up gradually. Pain is not used to guide the amount of activity. The hurt vs. harm explanation is utilized here. Surprisingly, many patients can increase their activity level substantially without a corresponding increase in pain after the first few days. This short-term discomfort is due to the use of muscles and joints that have been idle for a long time. A few patients use aspirin-like medication and mild muscle relaxants for the first week, but even these pain relievers are monitored closely to avoid fostering a dependence on any kind of medication to deal with pain.

By the time the patient has completed the program, he or she is able to do twenty minutes of aerobic exercise at a time, either on a stationary bicycle or a treadmill, and they should be able to do twenty repetitions of a series of activities prescribed for their individual needs. We attempt to simulate as closely as possible the movements the patient will have to perform at work and then we work on strengthening the muscles that will be needed for day-to-day activities. The physical and occupational therapists who are assigned full-time to the program assist with these activities. In addition some individualized therapies may be necessary, such as transcutaneous nerve stimulation.

4. *To improve coping skills.* To accomplish this goal, patients participate in group therapy five days a week, conducted by a clinical psychologist who guides them through a course of lectures on understanding pain and the psychological approaches to managing it. Individualized biofeedback may be provided for some patients, and individual counseling is made available when the team and psychiatric consultant find it appropriate. The patient's progress is monitored by weekly testing. Generally we see a lightening of depression, a decrease in anxiety, and a feeling of having more control over pain symptoms.

5. *To improve socialization and the enjoyment of recreational activities.* Our nurses and psychologists meet with patients, both in a group and alone. As needed, individual family sessions are held in which additional insights are provided to the patient's spouse and family members. We have found that when we include family members in the treatment program, the outcome is more successful and the results are maintained better—a conclusion paralleled by numerous national studies. But,

despite the fact that we strongly urge families to participate, only 30 to 50 percent seem to do so on a significant basis.

Assertiveness training is given through examples and education. The patients monitor their own recreational and social activities over the weekend by completing a questionnaire. This is reviewed on Monday to see which activities were attempted and how coping skills are improving. The recreational therapist sees the patients twice a week for outings. The patients themselves decide what they want to do and how to go about it. Under the close supervision of the therapist, patients may go shopping, to a movie, etc. A considerable amount of humor develops during these group activities.

6. *To return to work.* Helping our patients resume a productive life is an important goal of our program. Most are potentially employable, but at the time of admission, a significant number are unemployed and they feel very discouraged about their ability to return to work. Medical, legal, environmental, and work-related problems all may be standing in the way. We help with all facets of the vocational return, and the team works very closely with the employer and the insurance company to make this goal possible.

With some patients, the return to an eight-hour workday does not seem to be a reasonable goal, even with a very light level of activity. Some of these patients may have applied for social security disability or they may be on long-term disability. We work with these restrictions realistically.

Another percentage of patients is retired. The goal we have for them is to return to previous levels of independent functioning and enjoyment of their retirement years, with improved quality of life.

7. *To achieve graduation.* The big day comes when the patient is ready to be discharged from the Pain Rehabilitation Center. The decision is made at the Wednesday team conference and the patient is discharged on Friday of that week. We currently hold the graduation ceremony on the following Wednesday, and this is a special time for patients—they themselves usually make it a gala affair with poems, songs, and different pranks. Family and other people important to the patient are invited, and all the team members are present to bear witness to the patient's improvement. The graduates are presented with a certificate and they have the opportunity to express what they have achieved and how they did it. Usually they are very grateful to fellow patients who have helped them. As we stagger admissions, at any given time there might be two patients in their first week of the program, two patients in their second week, and two in their third week. Our senior patients are able to help the newcomers significantly.

8. *To support the patient with a good follow-up program.* Gains made in the pain program can be reversed quickly if adequate and continued support is lacking. All of our patients who finish the program are seen once a week for four weeks. The physician will examine the patient as needed. Any medication changes needed are made by the physician. Patients who have graduated are invited to share their experiences with patients still in the program. This has been a positive element contributing to the success of our program.

Three months after graduation the patients are reexamined by the whole team, and at this time, we perform our "program evaluation," a systematic measurement of the patient's success and the maintenance of that success. The information obtained is then compiled and analyzed to see whether the success is still being maintained.

One of the most important groups for patients in the Pain Rehabilitation Center is the *support group*. This group has met monthly since it was formed in 1985. The patients elect their own officers and put out a newsletter they call *Support Group Scoop*. The group gets together to provide ongoing education on advances in controlling chronic pain; to give mutual support in a therapeutic milieu to help maintain the gains made in the program; and to offer camaraderie and socialization. Many team members attend the meetings which are led by a nurse or a psychologist.

Since 1985, graduates have attended regularly and many have emphasized that they have been able to maintain control over their pain without using medications because of the support they have received in these meetings. In addition, these "senior" patients are a source of significant support and hope to more recent ones. It helps immeasurably to be able to look up to someone who is implementing the principles of the program successfully and working full-time.

At this writing, over 650 patients have been evaluated at the Pain Rehabilitation Center at Elmbrook Memorial Hospital. Over 500 of these have completed the program. Our follow-up indicates that all of our goals are being met by our patients at the end of the program. The goal achievements are being maintained after three months by over 85 percent of our patients. Over 70 percent of those who were unemployed when they entered the program have returned to work, but long-range studies are being continued.

The Center for Pain and
Work Rehabilitation (CPWR)

This program was established at St. Nicholas Hospital in Sheboygan, Wisconsin in 1991. Planning for it began in April 1991 and the first patients were accepted in November 1991. To date, over one hundred fifty patients have been evaluated and over ninety have gone through the comprehensive program.

As medical director, I worked closely in developing this program. CPWR is also a very comprehensive multidisciplinary program which closely matches the needs we have already described throughout this book. However, this is a purely outpatient program. If a patient has significant medication needs, dependence, depression, or has failed many outpatient approaches, they may be more successful in an inpatient setting.

However, if there are no major medication issues and the patient is willing to participate in the program, an outpatient program is a viable option.

The process of evaluation is performed by a physical therapist, psychologist and physician and includes a review of medical records. This is followed by a team conference, at which time a decision is made in regard to whether the patient needs to participate in the full program or can benefit from one of the individual components.

The program is four weeks in duration, and meets five days a week. On average, patients spend a minimum of five to six hours a week in education, physical and occupation therapy, nursing intervention and psychological group and individual sessions.

Early results of this program continue to reveal that a small community hospital can provide a comprehensive center for pain and work rehabilitation and be a major asset to the community.

Conclusion

This book emphasizes *your* personal ability to control pain. Pain is a personal experience. Only *you* know what type of pain it is and how significant it is to you. A physician must believe what the patient relates about pain, but the physician should use the best medical knowledge available to determine whether or not the symptom of pain is consistent with any underlying problem that can be treated with surgical, medical, physical, or psychiatric approaches. In those situations where a cure is not possible and the pain itself is leading to a significant disability, chronic pain management programs hold out much hope. Experiences over the last thirty years has shown that the chronic pain management program not only has been helpful, but that it is cost-effective when delivered in a rehabilitation model with the support of both patients and community.

RESOURCES

The following resources may be able to provide you with useful information.

ORGANIZATIONS

CARF

The Commission on Accreditation of Rehabilitation Facilities is a voluntary accrediting agency of rehabilitation programs in the country.

In 1982, CARF gathered together a national advisory committee to establish standards of chronic pain rehabilitation programs. I had the honor of being a member of the committee. Chronic pain standards were developed and became implemented in July, 1983. In 1987, a second national advisory committee was formed to update these standards, and once again, I served as a member. Unfortunately, at this time, CARF has standards for only comprehensive pain rehabilitation clinics. As I stated above, other types of pain clinics exist which provide valuable services to patients with acute or sub-acute types of pain problems. The medical community is beginning to identify the differences in these programs and provide them with appropriate accreditation. CARF can be contacted at 101 N. Wilmot Rd., Tuscon, AZ 85711 (800-444-8991).

AAPM

The American Academy of Pain Medicine (AAPM) is a national organization that is the official spokesmen for physicians who practice pain medicine. Formed in 1983 as the American Academy of Algology (AAA), members of this organization are physicians who have a major interest in the study and management of patients with chronic pain. Algo in Greek is pain, and logy is the science or study of.

The organization changed its name in 1987 to the American Academy of Pain Medicine. It currently has 650 members and conducts meetings annually to discuss not only the scientific elements of pain management, but its socioeconomic aspects as well. AAPM can be reached at 5700 Old Orchard Lane, Skokie, IL 60077 (708) 966-9510.

ACPM

The American College of Pain Medicine was established in June 1991, as an organization devoted to providing appropriate credentials through an examination process for physicians practicing pain medicine. The college is an independent organization that has developed a process for examination for those individuals who meet established criteria. This is an evolving area and the major goal of the college is to eventually assist in the recognition of "pain medicine" as a legitimate medical specialization area. In February 1993, the first ACPM examination was provided to over 100 qualified physicians. ACPM can be reached at 5700 Old Orchard Lane, Skokie, IL 60077 (708) 966-9510.

APS
American Pain Society is a multi-disciplinary organization which was formed in 1979. Its members include basic scientists and clinicians from a wide variety of backgrounds including physicians, psychologists, dentists, nurses, rehabilitation counselors, clinical and occupational therapists, social workers, and other health care professionals who are interested in the research and practice of pain medicine. There are over 2000 members in this organization. (708) 965-2776.

IPF
International Pain Foundation
909 NE 43rd St., Suite 306
Seattle, WA 98105
(206) 547-2157

SELF-HELP/OUTREACH

ACPA
American Chronic Pain Association
P.O. Box 850
Rocklin, CA 95677
(916) 632-0922

National Chronic Pain Outreach Association, Inc.
7979 Old Georgetown Rd., Suite 100
Bethesda, MD 20814-2429
(301) 652-4948

SHIP
(Self-help in Pain)
33 Kingadown Park
Whistable Kent C15 2DT
England UK

ACUTE PAIN

Pain Control after Surgery
Center for Research Dissemination/Liaison
AHCPR Publications
P.O. Box 8547
Silver Spring, MD 20907
(800) 358-9295

How to Talk to Your Doctor about Acute Pain
Du Pont Pharmaceuticals
Medical Products Department
Wilmington, DE 19898

ARTHRITIS

Arthritis
(General Information)
Arthritis Foundation
1314 Spring St. NW
Atlanta, GA 30309
(800) 283-7800

Arthritis
(Medicine for the Layman)
Public Inquiries Office
CC Building 10 Room 1C255
Bethesda, MD 20892

Arthritis—Coping with Pain
(The Battle Half Won)
Arthritis Foundation
1314 Spring St. NW
Atlanta GA 30309
(800) 283-7800

BACK PAIN

Preventing Backache
Health and Safety Unit
Metropolitan Insurance Company
1 Madison Avenue
New York, NY 10010

Taking Care of Your Back
American Physical Therapy Association
P.O. Box 37257
Washington, D.C. 20013

CANCER PAIN

Cancer Pain
(General information)
National Hospice Organization
1901 North Moore Street, Suite 901
Arlington, VA 22209
(800) 658-8898

Questions and Answers about Pain Control
(A Guide for People with Cancer and Their Families)
American Cancer Society
(800) 422-6237

Coping with Pain at Home
(A Guide for Cancer Patients and Their Families)
Du Pont Pharmaceuticals
Barley Mill Plaza, Bldg. 26
Wilmington, DE 19898

Cancer Pain Can Be Relieved
(A Guide for Patients and Families)
Wisconsin Cancer Pain Initiative
3675 Medical Sciences Center
University of Wisconsin
Madison, WI 53705

CHRONIC PAIN

Relieving Pain
Public Inquiries Office
Clinical Center
Bldg. 10, Room 1C255
Bethesda, MD 20892

Chronic Pain
(Hope Through Research)
Public Inquiries Office
National Institute of Neurological Disorders and Stroke
Bldg. 31, Room 8A06
Bethesda, MD 20892

Pain Research
(From Laboratory to Clinic)
Public Inquiries Office
P.O. Box 54793
Washington, D.C. 20032

Pain
(What Is It, How It Works, How We Cope with It)
Nuprin/Bristol Myers Company
P. O. Box 1000
Baltimore, MD 21268

FIBROMYALGIA

Fibromyalgia
(Fibrositis)
Arthritis Foundation
P. O. Box 19000
Atlanta, GA 30326

HEADACHE

Headache
(General Information)
National Headache Foundation
5252 North Western Avenue
Chicago, IL 60625
(312) 878-7715
(800) 843-2256

MEDICATIONS

Medicines and You
Office of Research Reports
National Institute of General Medical Sciences
Bldg. 31, Room 4A52
Bethesda, MD 20982
(301) 496-7301

REFLEX SYMPATHETIC DYSTROPHY

Reflex Sympathetic Dystrophy Syndrome Association
332 Haddon Avenue, Suite C
Westmont, NJ 08108
(609) 858-6553

SHINGLES

Shingles and Related Diseases
(The Fight Against VZV Infections)
The VZV Research Foundation Inc.
40 E. 72nd Street
New York, NY 10021
(212) 472-7148

Shingles
(Hope Through Research)
Public Inquiries Office
NINCDS
Bldg. 31, Room 8A06
Bethesda, MD 20892

Shingles
(What You Should Know)
Burroughs Wellcome Co.
Research Triangle Park
North Carolina, 27709

WOMEN

Pain and the Working Woman
Nuprin
Bristol Myers Company
P.O. Box 1000
Baltimore, MD 21268

JOURNALS

Pain. The journal of the International Association for the study of pain. Elseview, P.O. Box 321, 1000 AM Amsterdam, The Netherlands.

The Clinical Journal of Pain. Official journal of the American Academy of Pain Medicine. Raven Press, 1185 Avenue of America, New York, NY 10036.

Pain Digest. Ed. P.P. Raj. Springer-Verlag, 44 Hartz Way, Secaucus, NJ 07094.

Topics in Pain Management. Ed. J. Saper. Williams and Wilkins, 428 E. Preston St., Baltimore, MD 21202.

BIBLIOGRAPHY

SELF-HELP BOOKS

Abraham, Edward A. *Freedom from Back Pain*. (Rodale Press, 1986).

Arnold, Caroline. *Pain: What Is It? How Do We Deal With It?* (Morrow Junior Books, Morrow, 1986).

Catalano, Ellen Mohr. *The Chronic Pain Workbook*. (New Harbinger, 1987).

Fardon, F. *Stop the Pain*. (Price Stern, 1988).

Gil, Eliana. *Outgrowing the Pain*. (Dell, 1988).

Hendler, Nelson H., and Judith A. Fenton. *How to Cope With Chronic Pain*, revised edition, (Liberty, 1986).

Lawrence, Ronald M. *Goodbye Pain!* (Woodbridge Press, 1989).

Linchitz, Richard M. *Life Without Pain.* (Addison-Wesley, 1988).

Melzack, Ronald and Patrick Wall *The Challenge of Pain,* revised edition. (Penquin, 1989).

Ng, Lorenz K.Y. (Editor). *New Approaches to Treatment of Chronic Pain: A Review of Multidisciplinary Pain Clinics and Pain Centers.* NIDA Research Monograph #36. (Dept. of Health and Human Services, May 1981)

Olshan, Neal. *The Scottsdale Pain Relief Program: The Revolutionary Seven Day Drug-Free Program to Relieve Pain.* (Ballantine, 1988, Beaufort Books, 1987).

Sternbach, Richard A. *Mastering Pain.* (Ballantine, 1988; Putnam, 1987)

MEDICAL TEXTBOOKS

Abram, S. E. *The Pain Clinic Manual.* (J. B. Lippincott Co., Philadelphia, 1990).

Aronoff, G.M. *Evaluation and Management of Pain.* (Urban & Schwarzenberg, Baltimore, 1985).

Brena, S.F., Chapman, S.L. *Chronic Pain: Management Principles*. Clinics in Anesthesiology. (W.B. Saunders Co., Philadelphia, 1985).

Brena, S.F., Chapman, S.L. *Management of Patients with Chronic Pain*. (S.P. Medical and Scientific Books, New York, 1983).

Cailliet, R. *Soft Tissue Pain and Disability*. (F.A. Davis Company, Philadelphia, 1988).

Lynch, N.T., Vasudevan, S.V. *Persistent Pain: Psychosocial Assessment and Intervention*. (Kluwer Academic Publishers, Boston, 1988).

Portenoy, R.K. *Pain Mechanisms and Syndromes*. (W.B. Saunders Co., Philadelphia, 1989).

Stimmel, Barry. *Pain, Analgesia, and Addiction: The Pharmacological Treatment of Pain*. (Raven Press, New York, 1983).

Taylor, Humphrey, and Curran, Nancy Morency. *The Nuprin Pain Report*. (Louis Harris and Associates, Inc., New York, 1985).

Tollison, C. David. *Handbook of Chronic Pain Management*. (Williams and Wilkins, Baltimore, 1989).

Turk, D.C., Melzack, R. *Handbook of Pain Assessment*. (The Guilford Press, New York, 1992).

Background

SRIDHAR V. VASUDEVAN, M.D.

S ridhar V. Vasudevan, M.D., is clinical professor of Physical Medicine and Rehabilitation at the Medical College of Wisconsin in Milwaukee, Wisconsin. He is the Medical Director of the Pain Rehabilitation Center at Elmbrook Memorial Hospital in Brookfield, Wisconsin, and the Medical Director of the Center for Pain and Work Rehabilitation at St. Nicholas Hospital in Sheboygan, Wisconsin.

Dr. Vasudevan has over 15 years of experience in management of individuals with both acute and chronic pain. Dr. Vasudevan is past president of both the American Academy of Pain Medicine and the Midwest Pain Society. He is founding and past president of the

American College of Pain Medicine. He has been an active member and has served on the board of directors of the American Pain Society, an organization that represents the physicians and allied health professionals who are interested in pain management. He is also the past president of the Wisconsin Society of Physical Medicine and Rehabilitation.

Dr. Vasudevan has lectured extensively on the topic of pain rehabilitation at numerous medical conferences in the United States. In addition, he has spoken internationally at meetings in Scotland, Denmark, West Germany, India, Canada, the Peoples Republic of China, the Soviet Union, Australia, Mexico, and Israel. He has co-edited a text book on persistent pain and has authored numerous articles and chapters in several medical textbooks on the subject of pain and disability.

This book is based on experiences with programs designed to help individuals with chronic pain. It is aimed at patients (and their families) who have chronic pain or persistent pain, which essentially can control one's life. Through the principles presented in this book, the author hopes to provide these people with the knowledge and skills to take control over their pain, and eventually lead a productive and satisfying life.

STEPS TO
LIVING WITH PAIN

The following page lists the steps found in Chapter 9 which can be taken in learning to live with pain and find pleasure in life again. When you first try to manage your pain, you may need to read through these steps several times every day so that they are integrated into your daily life.

1. Accept the fact that you have chronic pain.

2. Set specific goals in your work, recreational, and social activities.

3. Direct your anger at the pain.

4. Stop taking all narcotic drugs.

5. Focus on achieving good physical health.

6. Learn relaxation techniques and then practice them.

7. Balance your activities. Learn to pace yourself.

8. Seek support—not sympathy, from your family, friends and co-workers.

9. Don't expect your doctor and the healthcare system to provide all the relief you seek.

10. Seek out experienced, supportive, professional help.

Adapted from *Mastering Pain: A Twelve-Step Program for Coping with Chronic Pain* by Dr. Richard A. Sternbach.

ORDER FORM

Please ship *Pain: A Four-Letter Word You Can Live With* to:

Name: _____
(Please print or type)

Address: _____
Street

_____
City   State   Zip

No. of books ordered ____ x $14.95 per book = $ _____

Wisconsin residents add 5% sales tax   _____

Milwaukee County residents add .5% sales tax   _____

Add $2.00 per book for shipping/handling   _____

Total Enclosed: $ _____

Please make checks payable to Montgomery Media, Inc.
Send this order form and your payment to:
    Pain: A Four-Letter Word You Can Live With
    Montgomery Media, Inc.
    611 N. Broadway, Suite 600
    Milwaukee, WI 53202

Discounts available for purchases of 10 books or more. For more information, write or call Montgomery Media, Inc., 611 N. Broadway, Suite 600, Milwaukee, Wisconsin 53202. (414) 223-4266.